Overcoming Insomnia

A Self-Help Guide Using Cognitive Behavioral Techniques

Colin A. Espie

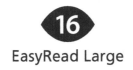

EasyRead Large

Copyright Page from the Original Book

Constable & Robinson Ltd
3 The Lanchesters
162 Fulham Palace Road
London W6 9ER
www.constablerobinson.com

First published in the UK by Robinson,
an imprint of Constable & Robinson Ltd, 2006

This edition published in 2010

Important Note
This book is not intended as a substitute for medical advice or treatment.
Any person with a condition requiring medical attention should consult a
qualified medical practitioner or suitable therapist.

ISBN: 978-1-84529-070-2

Typeset by TW Typesetting, Plymouth, Devon
Printed and bound in the EU

1 3 5 7 9 10 8 6 4 2

TABLE OF CONTENTS

Acknowledgements   v
Preface   vii
Introduction   ix
Foreword   xiv

PART ONE: Understanding Insomnia

Introduction to Part One   3
1: Normal sleep   4
2: Normal variations in sleep   31
3: Poor sleep and insomnia   50
4: The consequences of insomnia   74

PART TWO: Overcoming Insomnia and Becoming a Good Sleeper

Introduction to Part Two   93
5: Assessing your insomnia problem (Program Week 1)   98
6: Understanding sleep and insomnia (Program Week 2)   135
7: Sleep hygiene and relaxation (Program Week 3)   164
8: Scheduling a new sleep pattern(Program Week 4)   196
9: Dealing with a racing mind (Program Week 5)   220
10: Putting it all together (Program Week 6)   265

PART THREE: Special Circumstances

Introduction to Part Three   291
11: What about sleeping pills?   292
12: Recognizing and managing other common sleep
disorders   307

Glossary   333

Useful organizations   338

Further reading   342

Back Cover Material   347

Index   349

Colin Espie is Professor of Clinical Psychology and Director of the University of Glasgow Sleep Centre. He has published over 200 research papers on insomnia and is a leading member of the American Academy of Sleep Medicine and the European Sleep Research Society.

The aim of the **Overcoming** series is to enable people with a range of common problems and disorders to take control of their own recovery program. Each title, with its specially tailored program, is devised by a practising clinician using the latest techniques of cognitive behavioral therapy – techniques which have been shown to be highly effective in changing the way patients think about themselves and their difficulties. The series was initiated in 1993 by Peter Cooper, Professor of Psychology at Reading University in the UK, whose original volume on overcoming bulimia nervosa and binge-eating continues to help many people in the USA, UK, Europe and Australasia.

Other titles in the series include:

OVERCOMING ANGER AND IRRITABILITY
OVERCOMING ANOREXIA NERVOSA
OVERCOMING ANXIETY
OVERCOMING BODY IMAGE PROBLEMS
OVERCOMING BULIMIA NERVOSA AND
BINGE-EATING
OVERCOMING CHILDHOOD TRAUMA
OVERCOMING CHRONIC FATIGUE
OVERCOMING CHRONIC PAIN
OVERCOMING COMPULSIVE GAMBLING
OVERCOMING DEPERSONALIZATON AND
FEELINGS OF UNREALITY

OVERCOMING DEPRESSION
OVERCOMING GRIEF
OVERCOMING HEALTH ANXIETY
OVERCOMING LOW SELF-ESTEEM
OVERCOMING MOOD SWINGS
OVERCOMING OBSESSIVE COMPULSIVE
DISORDER
OVERCOMING PANIC
OVERCOMING PARANOID AND SUSPICIOUS
THOUGHTS
OVERCOMING PROBLEM DRINKING
OVERCOMING RELATIONSHIP PROBLEMS
OVERCOMING SEXUAL PROBLEMS
OVERCOMING SOCIAL ANXIETY AND SHYNESS
OVERCOMING STRESS
OVERCOMING TRAUMATIC STRESS
OVERCOMING WEIGHT PROBLEMS
OVERCOMING WORRY
OVERCOMING YOUR CHILD'S FEARS AND
WORRIES
OVERCOMING YOUR CHILD'S SHYNESS AND
SOCIAL ANXIETY
OVERCOMING YOUR SMOKING HABIT

All titles in the series are available by mail
order.
Please see the order form at the back of this
book.
www.overcoming.co.uk

To Aud: my wife and my soulmate

Acknowledgements

I would like to thank a number of people who have made a major contribution, in various ways, to the work underlying this book. There are far too many to mention by name, but I hope that by summarizing I can adequately reflect my very sincere gratitude.

First of all I am grateful to the many research colleagues I have known and worked with over the years in Canada, the USA, Australia, Europe and, of course, in the UK. The development and evaluation of CBT for insomnia has been, and continues to be, an international effort, and I have been privileged to be part of that work. Then there is my own research team at the University of Glasgow Sleep Research Laboratory; both current members of my group and those that have worked with me across the years. Scores of highly motivated research fellows, research assistants, research nurses, postgraduates and administrative staff have helped to keep the show on the road. More than that – these people have been the lifeblood of my professional life.

My personal assistant Anita McClelland deserves special thanks, not only for her typing of the drafts of this book, but also for putting up with me over the past ten years! Every productive professional has a good administrator in the background, and I would like to thank Anita for always being there to help.

None of this, of course, would have been possible without our patients and research participants, from whom we find out, through one research method or another, everything that we know about the perplexing yet intriguing disorder that we call 'insomnia'.

Finally, I have a wonderful and supportive family of whom I am immensely proud: Craig, who is fulfilling his father's alternative dream by studying and playing music; Carolyn, who is following in our footsteps through her studies in psychology; and our youngest, Robbie, who at five years of age is already able to take charge of most of life's major decisions! Most of all, there is my alluring and very special wife, Audrey, to whom I dedicate this book with all my love.

Preface

I am writing this preface while on sabbatical leave at Université Laval, Québec City. I had promised myself that the book would be finished around four weeks ago, but I guess to be only a month behind schedule for an undertaking of this size is not so bad. Anyway, that's life, is it not?

The priorities and pressures are such that most of us in academic life spend the majority of our time conducting research, analyzing data, writing scientific papers, and teaching our students. Those of us who are clinical academics also try to fit in seeing the occasional patient or two. In this context, writing books for the general public is at best regarded as a hobby; at worst even a misuse of our time. Yet what is the purpose of knowledge if it is not to share it, and to try to improve things for people?

I struggled with this dilemma for a while. However, I decided last year, after being approached by the publishers, that the time had finally come to 'do the book!' I am sure that other authors in the excellent CBT series that Constable and Robinson produce have probably felt the same way. I guess most of us have a lay readership book in us. Well for better or for worse this one is mine.

It has actually felt very good writing the book. It has given me the opportunity to make available to you the treatment materials that we have developed and evaluated in our research studies. That feels like the right thing to do. What you are getting here is pretty much a complete CBT treatment guide for insomnia; the way I would present it to you if you came to my clinic in Glasgow. Of course, I can't get the particular 'angles' that are special to you and to your sleep problems. However, that said, I am confident that you have a very powerful tool in your hands that will help you towards overcoming your insomnia.

I wish you success as you set out on this course of CBT treatment. Sleep soundly and sleep well.

Colin A. Espie
BSc, MAppSci, PhD, FBPsS,
CPsychol Université Laval,
Québec City, Canada

Introduction

Why a cognitive behavioral approach?

You may have picked up this book uncertain as to why a psychological approach, such as a cognitive behavioral one, might help you overcome your sleep problems. A brief account of the history of this form of treatment might be helpful and encouraging. In the 1950s and 1960s a set of therapeutic techniques was developed, collectively termed 'behavior therapy'. These techniques shared two basic features. First, they aimed to remove symptoms (such as anxiety) by dealing with those symptoms themselves, rather than their deep-seated, underlying historical causes (traditionally the focus of psychoanalysis, the approach developed by Sigmund Freud and his associates). Second, they were loosely related to what laboratory psychologists were discovering about the mechanisms of learning, and could potentially be put to the test, or had already been proven to be of practical value to sufferers. The area where these techniques proved to be of most value was in the treatment of anxiety disorders, especially specific phobias (such as extreme fear of animals or heights), notoriously difficult to treat using conventional psychotherapies.

After an initial flush of enthusiasm, discontent with behavior therapy grew. There were a number of reasons for this, an important one was the fact that behavior therapy did not deal with the internal thoughts which were so obviously central to the distress that many patients were experiencing. In particular, behavior therapy proved inadequate when it came to the treatment of depression. In the late 1960s and early 1970s a treatment for depression was developed called 'cognitive therapy'. The pioneer in this enterprise was an American psychiatrist, Professor Aaron T. Beck. He developed a theory of depression which emphasized the importance of people's depressed styles of thinking, and, on the basis of this theory, he specified a new form of therapy. It would not be an exaggeration to say that Beck's work has changed the nature of psychotherapy, not just for depression but for a range of psychological problems.

The techniques introduced by Beck have been merged with the techniques developed earlier by the behavior therapists to produce a therapeutic approach which has come to be known as 'cognitive behavioral therapy' (CBT). This therapy has been subjected to the strictest scientific testing and it has been found to be a highly successful treatment for a significant proportion of cases of depression. It has now become clear that specific patterns of disturbed thinking are associated with a wide range of psychological problems, not just depression, and that the treatments which deal with these are highly effective. So, effective cognitive behavioral treatments have been developed for anxiety disorders, like panic disorder, generalized anxiety disorder, specific phobias and social phobia, obsessive compulsive disorders, and hypochondriasis (health anxiety), as well as for other conditions such as compulsive gambling, drug addiction, and eating disorders like bulimia nervosa. Indeed, cognitive behavioral techniques have been found to have a wide application beyond the narrow categories of psychological disorders. They have been applied effectively, for example, to helping people with low self-esteem, those with marital difficulties or weight problems, those who wish to give up smoking or excessive drinking, and, as in this book, those with sleep problems.

The starting-point for CBT is the realization that the ways we think, feel and behave are all intimately linked, and changing the way we think about ourselves, our experiences, and the world around us changes the way we feel and what we are able to do. So, for example, by helping a depressed person identify and challenge their automatic depressive thoughts, a route out of the cycle of depressive thoughts and feelings can be found. Similarly, habitual behavioral responses are driven by a complex set of thoughts and feelings, and CBT, as you will discover from this book, by providing a means for the behavior to be brought under cognitive control, enables these responses to be undermined and a different kind of life to be possible.

Although effective CBT treatments have been developed for a wide range of disorders and problems, these treatments are not widely available; and, when people try to help themselves on their own, they often do things which make matters worse. In recent years the community of cognitive behavioral therapists has responded to this situation. What they have done is to take the principles and techniques of specific cognitive behavioral therapies for particular problems and present them in manuals, which people can read and apply themselves. These manuals specify a systematic program of treatment which the individual works through to overcome their difficulties. In this way, cognitive behavioral therapeutic techniques of proven value are being made available on the widest possible basis.

Self-help manuals are never going to replace therapists. Many people will need individual treatment from a qualified therapist. It is also the case that, despite the widespread success of CBT, some people will not respond to it and will need one of the other treatments available. Nevertheless, although research on the use of these self-help manuals is at an early stage, the work done to date indicates that for a great many people such a manual will prove sufficient for them to overcome their problems without professional help. Many people suffer silently and secretly for years. Sometimes appropriate help is not forthcoming, despite their efforts to find it.

Sometimes they feel too ashamed or guilty to reveal their problems to anyone. For many of these people the cognitive behavioral self-help manual will provide a lifeline to recovery and a better future.

Professor Peter Cooper
The University of Reading, 2005

Foreword

To be unable to sleep is one of life's worst experiences. Insomnia not only affects your night-time, through disrupted and unsatisfactory sleep, but it also has consequences in terms of your quality of life. People with persistent sleep problems of this type often complain of being slowed down mentally or moody during the day. What is more, they are not the only ones who suffer. Broken sleep can affect partners, children, and our social life and working life.

Insomnia is a major public health problem. Billions of dollars are spent worldwide every year on prescribed medications, over-the-counter remedies, and other suggested solutions – all in the search of a decent sleep. One in ten adults, and one in five of those over 65 years of age, have insomnia. Being unable to sleep is one of the most common complaints heard by doctors, yet our healthcare systems are barely scratching the surface in offering a service that will help people.

Research conducted over the past 25 years has established cognitive behavioral therapy (CBT) as an effective treatment for persistent insomnia. Indeed, leading authorities now regard CBT as the treatment of first choice. But there is a problem – CBT is not widely available because clinical psychology services and behavioral medicine services do not have the capacity at this time to meet the potential demand. These are professions that are, in relative terms, still in their infancy. So, while the research has been conducted and the evidence is there, the means to deliver CBT is lagging behind.

As one of the people who has been most closely involved with the development and evaluation of insomnia treatment, I want to help you make the best possible use of the CBT program that we have developed in Scotland. I believe that one of the ways to help overcome the scale of the insomnia problem that is out there is to put the solution, the CBT itself, directly into your hands. We as professionals must, and will, continue to lobby politicians and healthcare providers to develop much-needed services. However, there is also a lot that you can do to improve your sleep yourself, if you are given the right tools for the job.

This book is designed for your use as a CBT treatment manual. I have set out the different parts of the book, and the chapters within each part, so that you can use it as a CBT self-help program. You are about to set out on a course of therapy. I will be your therapist, as it were from a distance, but you must take on the role not only of patient but also of co-therapist. You will be learning and implementing at the same time ... you will be evaluating your own progress ... you will get what you give! Like any course of treatment, I ask you to take this CBT program seriously. Give it some of your best-quality time and attention.

In our studies evaluating the effectiveness of CBT we have seen a great many patients who thought they would never be able to sleep well, go on to make huge improvements in the pattern and the quality of their sleep. CBT offers you this prospect. Join me in helping you benefit ... let's overcome insomnia together!

PART ONE

Understanding Insomnia

Introduction to Part One

The first part of the book is about developing an understanding of sleep and of insomnia. I hope you will find that this is a helpful step towards your goal of learning how to overcome insomnia and how to become a good sleeper. Try not to be tempted to jump ahead to Part Two, especially if you are the kind of person who likes to 'get on with it'! Part One will give you important background information that will make it much easier to put your cognitive behavioral treatment into practice.

1

Normal sleep

What is sleep?

You may be surprised by this, but I would like to begin by explaining what sleep is *not.* This is important, because sleep is very commonly misunderstood.

First, sleep is *not* simply the absence of wakefulness. Falling asleep is not like having a light switched off, just as wakefulness is not the same as a light switched on. The on/off idea would suggest that we live our lives either at one extreme or the other. This is not in fact correct, because there are variations within sleep, just as there are variations in wakefulness. You are not always 'wide awake' ... are you? Similarly, you are not always 'fast asleep'.

Second, sleep is *not* an inactive process. Sleep is not 'down tools' time, or a kind of respite or escape. On the contrary, the body's activities during sleep are absolutely vital to life. Your sleep is a part of your life, not something separate from it – you have heard it said that we spend one-third of our lives asleep (I hear you say 'I wish!'). Just because we are unconscious, and have no memory for the greater part of our sleep, does not mean that sleep is either a simple or a passive state.

So what then *is* sleep? The famous Israeli scientist Dr Peretz Lavie once wrote a semi-autobiographical book about his experiences in sleep research. He called the book *TheEnchanted World of Sleep.* For me this title captures the fact that sleep is rich, diverse, and precious; and still fascinatingly mysterious. We live our lives not just in the waking world. Let's go and take a glimpse at life within sleep.

Research studies have shown us that sleep is a very complex, yet very ordered process. Scientists have discovered the exity of sleep by studying the activity of the brain during sleep-laboratory recordings. Sleep is made up of different subtypes and stages. Sleep is also orderly, because these types and stages of sleep are organized in a series of cycles that repeat across the night.

Sleep is also active in other ways. For example, it is during sleep that our body tissue is repaired. Proteins, the building-blocks of life, are laid down during sleep, and some hormones are produced selectively during the night, such as the growth hormone in developing infants and children. So there is some truth in the idea that we grow during the night! These are just a few examples of physical processes that occur during sleep, but there are also very important mental processes. We catch a glimpse of this in the phenomenon of dreaming. Of course, we do not always remember our dreams, but when we do what is very apparent is that we have been thinking, even while we were asleep. Enchanting!

Measuring sleep in the laboratory

In order to understand this complex process it may be helpful to find out a little about how sleep is 'measured' and analyzed; this is usually done in a *sleep laboratory.*

Scientists study sleep by taking three types of measurement:

1 Electrical activity in the brain is measured by *electroencephalography* (EEG). This measure is used because the EEG signals associated with being awake are different from those found during sleep. Also, the different stages of sleep can be measured using EEG.

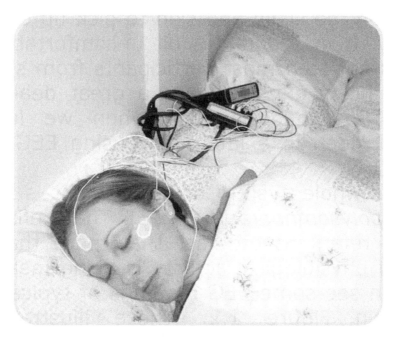

Figure 1.1 A typical sleep laboratory assessment taking place

2 Muscle activity is measured using *electromyography* (EMG), because muscle tone also differs between wakefulness and sleep. Once again, there are EMG differences within sleep, depending upon the stage of sleep.

3 Third, eye movements during sleep are measured using *electro-oculography* (EOG). This is a very specific measurement that helps to identify dreaming sleep. The eyeballs make characteristic movements that show us when someone is in this type of sleep.

Figure 1.1 shows a typical sleep assessment taking place. Electrodes are placed at various points on the scalp and skin to pick up electrical activity. It may sound a bit uncomfortable, but it does not stop most participants from sleeping and it helps experts learn a great deal about sleep. So what happens when we look at normal sleep in a laboratory using EEG, EMG, and EOG?

This whole system of assessment is usually called *polysomnography* (PSG). The prefix 'poly' simply refers to the fact that more than one type of physiological activity is being measured. You can see some EEG readings of typical adult sleep in Figure 1.2. These illustrate the similarities and differences between the different stages of sleep. You can also make some comparisons of sleep with waking.

The stages of sleep

Let's start with waking. Sometimes we call this *Stage W* (wakefulness). You will see that the EEG part of the tracing is characterized by what we call 'fast activity'. EEG waves are fairly random and of low voltage. You will see in Figure 1.2 that they are of relatively low height *(amplitude)* and are generated in close proximity to one another *(high frequency)*. Waking EEG of this type is known as *beta* activity. Notice next the difference between this EEG and the one depicted in the third row in Figure 1.2. This is an EEG of someone in bed with their eyes closed, and you can see that the EEG waves no longer come quite as thick or fast. This is what is called *alpha* activity or *alpha* rhythm.

As we fall asleep we go into a transitional phase between wakefulness and sleep known as *Stage 1* sleep. Compared with quiet wakefulness, the EEG waves in Stage 1 slow down to around three to seven cycles per second (cps). These are known as *theta* waves.

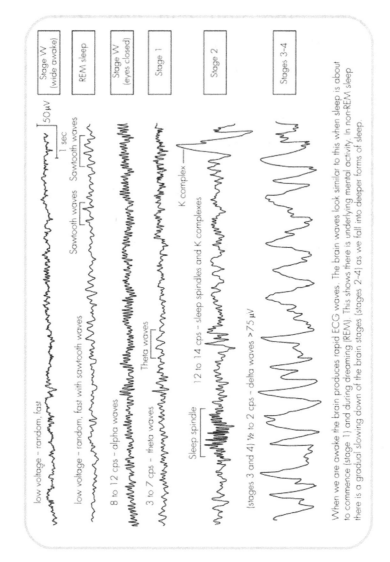

Figure 1.2 A polysomnographic (PSG) recording showing the different stages of sleep

Figure 1.2 shows only the EEG for Stage 1 sleep, but if you were to see a measurement for muscle tone (EMG) during Stage 1, you would notice that the muscles begin to relax in comparison with wakefulness. Similarly, the EOG traces would change and begin to show slow *rolling eye movements.* Stage 1 sleep normally lasts only a matter of minutes before progressing to Stage 2.

You can see that the EEG varies considerably during *Stage 2* sleep. There are *mixed frequencies* of EEG waves (some fast, some slow, some high amplitude, some low). However, there are two characteristic formations that occur repeatedly, and these are the defining features of Stage 2 sleep. The *K-complex* takes its name from the shape of an initially descending and then ascending sharp change in voltage. By tradition lines on the upward inclination in EEGs are called 'descending' and those heading downward are called 'ascending' – this may seem odd, but it is the standard terminology. The other features of Stage 2 sleep are known as *sleep spindles* – the name for rapid bursts of high-frequency EEG activity (12–14cps) that occur intermittently. Although Stage 2 sleep comprises the largest proportion of adult sleep (50–60 per cent), the first phase of Stage 2 sleep is usually quite short.

We have the deepest part of our sleep during the first third of the night, and there is a more rapid transition into *deep sleep* during this period. EEG *Stage 3* and *Stage 4* together make up this deep sleep, sometimes called *slow-wave sleep* because the EEG now reveals higher waves occurring at much lower frequencies. The height of these *delta waves* will be 75 microvolts (µV) or greater, and the wave frequency has now dropped to its lowest at 1/2–2cps. The difference between Stages 3 and 4 is simply the proportion of each 30-second period of sleep analysis during which delta waves are present. For Stage 3 sleep, 20–50 per cent comprises delta waves, whereas more than 50 per cent is required for describing sleep as Stage 4. Deep sleep is a form of *synchronized sleep* because the brain's electrical activity settles to a harmonized rhythm, and so produces the steady 'beats' that you can see in Figure 1.2.

So far, then, we can see that the transition from wakefulness through to deep sleep involves not only a loss of consciousness, but also a steady change in the EEG wave pattern from fast to slow activity, and that four stages of sleep can be differentiated. However, in 1953 two researchers in Chicago, Dr Kleitman and his young assistant Dr Aserinsky, made a crucial discovery about sleep. They noticed that there was another form of sleep during which the eyeballs move rapidly, whereas the rest of the body is pretty much paralyzed. The term *rapid eye movement (REM) sleep* was coined, and so important was its discovery that all the other Stages (1, 2, 3, and 4) actually became known as non-REM sleep.

You can see in Figure 1.2 that the EEG during REM sleep does not look very different from wakefulness or from Stage 1 sleep.

Indeed, it is a form of light sleep. However, the EOG shows very characteristic eye movements, and the EMG shows a marked flattening (loss of muscle tone). This actually makes sense when you think that it is during REM sleep that we do most of our dreaming. Were it not for the fact that our major voluntary muscles are relaxed, we could easily injure ourselves by acting out our dreams! You may not have realized before that you are in fact very still in your bed during your dreams, in spite of whatever vivid dream imagery you may experience. Occasional muscle twitches are quite usual, but any movement on a large scale during REM sleep is uncommon. In fact, if this does occur it may mean that the person has a problem known as *REM sleep behavior disorder.* This is not the same as *sleepwalking,* which occurs during periods of non-REM deep sleep. I will explain more about the different disorders of sleep later in this book.

Evaluating a sleep recording

Sleep records from the sleep laboratory are *scored* by highly trained professionals into the different stages of sleep. Sometimes we call this process *staging sleep.* We still use a standard set of scoring rules developed in the USA in the late 1960s by Dr Rechtschaffen and Dr Kales. In the early days, information from each recording channel (EEG, EMG, EOG) was printed out and reviewed page by page. Nowadays this information is analyzed on a PC screen and the person doing the scoring scrolls through, allocating each 30-second chunk, or *epoch,* to one of the sleep stages.

After a sleep recording has been scored, the computer generates a *sleep report.* This summarizes the night and provides useful information for the researcher to work with. An example of an abbreviated sleep report from my own lab can be seen in Figure 1.3. Let me take you through the information presented there.

You can see that the report begins with *record identification* information about the patient. Obviously we do not want to give away any confidential details, so we have called this 50-year-old man John Smith, and given him a made-up date of birth. He has a diagnosis of 'psychophysiologic insomnia' and has had persistent sleep problems for the past 12 years. You are going to hear a lot more about this type of insomnia later in this book. Each patient is given a unique sleep study code, and his or her hospital number or research protocol number would usually be included. Here you will see the file name is simply made up from this sample patient's name, the lab bedroom he slept in (lab 2), and the night of his stay (night 3).

Next there is a section of the report headed *sleep parameters.* You can see that we use the standard 30-second epoch length for scoring sleep stages. John Smith's bedtime was recorded as 10:50p.m. and his rising time as 7:21a.m. This means that his time in bed (TIB) was just over 8 1/2 hours, at 511 minutes. However, he did not sleep for 8 1/2 hours! As you can see, John Smith has a severe insomnia problem.

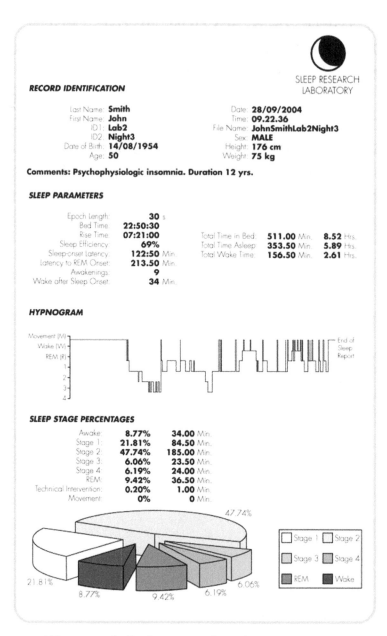

Figure 1.3 A sample sleep report

We use the term *sleep-onset latency (SOL)* for the length of time it takes someone to fall asleep. Here the SOL is 122 minutes, so it took John Smith more than 2 hours to get to sleep on this particular night. As well as the time taken to get off to sleep, we are interested in whether or not there were problems staying asleep. This report contains two pieces of information about the continuity of John Smith's sleep. You can see that nine *awakenings* from sleep were recorded. *Wake time after sleep-onset (WASO)* is the total amount of time spent awake during these awakenings. Here the WASO was 34 minutes, so we can work out that John Smith's wakeful episodes were relatively brief. Nevertheless, these can be quite disruptive because they impair sleep quality. If you think about it, together SOL and WASO represent the most common insomnia complaints: difficulty getting to sleep, and difficulty staying asleep. John Smith's *total wake time (TWT)* was 156 minutes.

Of course, we also want to know how much sleep John Smith obtained. You can see, therefore, that his *total sleep time (TST)* amounted to 5 hours and 53 minutes.

The sleep parameters section also includes information on something called *sleep efficiency (SE).* This is an important figure because it tells us the proportion (percentage) of the time in bed that was spent asleep. It is calculated as TST/TIB x 100. In this example, total sleep time (TST) was 353 minutes out of the 511 minutes of time in bed (TIB), so the SE was 69 per cent; a pretty poor night by any standards! Generally, we think of an SE below 85 per cent as being a potential problem, and above 85 per cent as being good sleep. This of course raises the interesting point that it is not necessarily *how much sleep* we get that is important, but *how good a quality* it is. Sleeping through for 6 continuous hours from lights out to waking would give an SE of 100 per cent, whereas getting a total of 6 hours broken up over an 8-hour period would give an SE of only 75 per cent. You will find out later that improving your sleep efficiency is one of the key requirements in overcoming insomnia.

We now move on to the *hypnogram* and the sleep stage percentages. The hypnogram gives us a picture of John Smith's sleep pattern across the night, throughout the different stages of sleep. You can see, for example, that his awakenings generally happened in the second half of the night. The sleep report gives us the *percentage* of the night spent in each stage of sleep (1, 2, 3, 4, REM). Over half the night was spent in Stage 2 sleep, with a further 24 per cent in Stage 1. As I explained earlier, Stage 1 sleep is a transitional form of sleep that normally makes up a relatively small percentage of our total time asleep.

John Smith's total slow-wave or deep sleep can be calculated by adding together his sleep Stages 3 and 4. This amounts to only 47 minutes, or around 13 per cent of the night. So we can deduce that John Smith must be quite a light sleeper.

Looking back to the sleep parameters, you can also see that his *latency to REM onset* – that is, how long it was before the first episode of REM sleep occurred – was 213 minutes on this particular night. This is much longer than we normally find on a good night's sleep, when 60–70 minutes would be more usual. John Smith spent a total of 36 minutes in REM, about half what we would expect to see in a man of his age. Finally, you can see that the report contains sleep stage information on Stage W, and another category, *movement time (M),* which we use if it is not possible to decide on a sleep or wake stage. This might be when the EEG channels are impossible to read. In John Smith's case this measurement wasn't necessary, though there was a brief *technical intervention* (perhaps checking an electrode) by one of our staff.

Before leaving this topic I want to take a moment to consider whether or not people sleep normally in a sleep laboratory. You might be thinking that with all this equipment attached, your sleep continuity and sleep quality might be quite different ... and of course there's the added element of being in a strange environment. Dr Jack Edinger from the VA Medical Center, Durham and Duke University, North Carolina, has completed a number of important studies investigating home versus lab-based sleep-assessment (polysomnography, or PSG) in insomnia. His findings are interesting because they suggest that it might be better if sleep could be measured at home, because in a lab setting people can actually sleep *better* than usual. In part this could be due simply to the change of environment. Another possibility is that they might not *expect* to be able to sleep in a lab, and those lower expectations could mean that they are less anxious about sleep, and so sleep better. This research work, then, also introduces us to one of the psychological components of insomnia – the importance of expectations!

On the experience of sleep

You have probably never been to a sleep laboratory, but I am sure you have tried to measure your sleep somehow – perhaps by working out how long you think you have slept, or how long it took you to fall asleep, or how many times you woke up during the night. These are measures of the *experience of sleep,* of what you remember about your sleep, and of the conclusions that you draw about your sleep. I bet you have found that it is not easy to calculate these things very accurately.

You may even have tried to keep some type of *Sleep Diary* so that you can see what your sleep is like over a period of time, or to try to work out if there is a pattern. Diaries like this are very useful, and we will be using them quite a bit as we assess and treat your insomnia. What I am saying is that your experience of sleep is *very important,* because that is what you have been living with.

Sometimes it is easier to think about the quality of our sleep rather than its quantity. *Sleep quality* and sleep efficiency have something in common. For example, you might feel that you have had a 'good sleep' or a 'deep sleep' – or, perhaps more likely because you are reading this book, that you have had many nights of 'restless sleep' or 'hardly any sleep', or that it takes you a long time to get into a proper sleep. It's not always easy to convert these kinds of experience into numbers. Whether we are trying to estimate quantity or commenting on sleep quality, this is called *subjective assessment.* But we should not fall into the trap of thinking that subjective assessment is less important than the objective kind (as is done in sleep clinics). What you think and feel about your sleep is extremely important, not least because it is your experience of sleep (or lack of sleep) that usually makes you seek help in the first place.

It is likely that it was your experience of poor sleep that led you to be interested in this book in the first place. So it will be important for you to keep accurate records of your subjective sleep experiences, and I will help you make best use of a Sleep Diary. This form of assessment is recognized internationally as *essential* for clinical work in insomnia. In other words, the experience of insomnia, systematically summarized on a night-to-night basis, is the most important thing in eventually treating it.

There are different sub-types of insomnia, and we will be learning more about these in Chapter 3. One of the more common ones is *psychophysiologic insomnia.* In this form of insomnia, the person's experience of sleep can be confirmed by objective measurements such as PSG. In other words, someone with psychophysiologic insomnia may estimate that on a given night it took 45 minutes to get to sleep, and assessment will confirm that they had difficulty getting off to sleep. Similarly, if the problem was staying asleep (a sleep maintenance problem), both objective tests and self-reports will tend to agree.

However, you may be already familiar with the common finding from research that people usually sleep longer than they think they have done. Research literature tells us that people with insomnia tend to overestimate how long it takes them to fall asleep (SOL), how long they are awake during the night (WASO), and their total amount of sleep (TST). This has been taken by some to mean that people with insomnia 'exaggerate' their problem. Little wonder that many people with insomnia feel that their complaints are not taken seriously. However, this *discrepancy* should not surprise us. People who are normally good sleepers are likely to make very similar 'errors' in estimation on those occasional nights when they sleep poorly. This suggests to me that it is not so much the person with insomnia who is in some way at fault, rather that the task is actually quite a hard one, and one that good sleepers seldom have to perform. During the night, in the absence of stimulation and activity, time can appear to pass rather slowly (don't you know it!).

Another possibility has some support from recent research on insomnia carried out by Dr Michael Perlis at the University of Rochester in New York State. This work suggests that sleep assessment (PSG), when scored in the conventional way into sleep stages, may fail to identify more subtle EEG characteristics that form part of the underlying pattern in insomnia. For example, a tendency towards waking up very, very briefly, or the presence of fast EEG waves (as in wakefulness or light sleep) intruding into sleep, may correspond better to subjective experiences of insomnia. In other words, we may in time need to study sleep using a different set of criteria. Much more research in this area is required.

But I never slept a wink!

'Oh yes, you did,' you will have heard; 'Oh no, I didn't' you may have answered, or felt like answering! Hopefully, the sections above can help you understand how differences can arise in the way people perceive sleep. There is, however, a particular form of insomnia where the hallmark feature is this debate, or I might even say dispute, about whether or not sleep actually occurred.

Clinicians and researchers have come to recognize a disorder that used to be called, until very recently, *sleep-state misperception.* In this type of insomnia the individual remains convinced that he or she obtained no or hardly any sleep, often over many years. On the one hand this seems unlikely, but on the other hand there can be no doubt that these beliefs are sincerely held, by perfectly sensible and reasonable people.

When this disorder has been studied in the laboratory, sleep patterns that are fairly normal are often found. How can this be? Well, perhaps these are extreme cases of the disparity between different methods of assessment; the 'subjective–objective discrepancy'. But we might just as accurately conclude that assessments such as PSG are simply not up to capturing the nature of this type of sleep experience. For these reasons, this disorder has now been given the name *paradoxical insomnia,* to reinforce the paradoxical nature of the problem: apparently sleeping well yet complaining of severe insomnia. Paradoxical insomnia should be a priority for further research, and I feel strongly that this diagnosis should not be misused to criticize people who have such symptoms.

Let us never forget, then, that a person's individual experience of sleep may be different from the sleep records obtained in a sleep lab. Both are important, and they are not necessarily in competition with one another for 'right' and 'wrong'. We need to recognize that concern about insomnia is what brings people to the attention of health services. Without that, no help will be offered, or needed. I am sure that time, and good science, will tell that there are better laboratory measures yet to come.

What controls our sleep pattern?

Two processes are commonly recognized as working together to regulate our sleep pattern. One is called the *sleep homeostat,* and this controls our 'drive' for sleep; the other is called the *circadian timer,* and controls *when* we sleep.

Broadly speaking, the longer we are awake, the sleepier we will become. Extended wakefulness, therefore, increases the body's drive for sleep. In physiology, this kind of process is there to restore balance, so sleep reduces the drive for sleep, and wakefulness increases the sleep drive, in much in the same way that we become parched if we go without fluids, and drinking satisfies that thirst and so reduces the drive to drink.

The famous sleep researcher Dr William C. Dement from Stanford University, California, uses the helpful analogy of the 'sleep economy'. With each hour that we spend awake we accumulate an increasing *sleep debt.* In healthy good sleepers this debt is repaid in full by the night's sleep and they awaken refreshed and back 'in balance' the next morning. The analogy raises the possibility that there are individuals who, perhaps through lifestyle choices or for other reasons, find themselves in a state of chronic sleep debt. Indeed, there may be attitudes within some parts of modern society that encourage such lifestyles and pay scant attention to nature's way of replenishing and restoring the body. The drive for sleep is, naturally, stronger when we first go to bed than it is later on, and this accounts, for example, for why it is that a nap can make us feel much better. Similarly, some people report waking after a couple of hours of sleep and feeling quite awake and refreshed. It is also a reason, of course, to *avoid* napping if you have insomnia, because naps have the potential to reduce the body's drive for sleep during the night, when you really want it to work for you.

You may have heard of the *circadian rhythm.* This is a term used to describe the harmony of the sleep–wake schedule. Other functions apart from sleep, such as body temperature, also follow recognized circadian patterns. We are designed to function in a 24-hour world. The word 'circadian' derives from the Latin words *circa diem,* literally meaning 'around the day'. Sometimes we talk about the *body clock,* meaning pretty much the same thing.

Our circadian rhythm takes a little while to become established. During early development an infant's sleep is not organized into day and night phases. Instead, babies sleep and wake across the 24 hours. By around 6 months, however, the major sleep period becomes concentrated and more settled during the night-time hours of darkness, there is more wakefulness during daytime/daylight hours, and the body clock gradually approximates to local time. The hormone *melatonin* is largely responsible for the ongoing regulation of the body clock throughout our lives. Melatonin is produced in the brain, in the *pineal gland.* Its production rate is dictated by natural light, so that during hours of darkness (the normal sleep period) melatonin production increases, and as morning approaches and with the coming of daylight, melatonin production is once again shut down. Of course there is some natural variation in circadian alertness during the daytime. For example, you will probably be aware of the *afternoon dip* when we tend to feel temporarily rather more tired. Indeed, in some societies it is normal to have a siesta at this time because it also coincides with the hottest part of the day. In terms of our circadian tendencies there is much to be said for that lifestyle!

Before moving on from this section, however, it is important to note that it is the *interaction* of the sleep homeostat and the circadian timing mechanism that, under normal circumstances, leads to good sleep. This is when the drive for sleep becomes strongest during normal hours of darkness, and results in an absence of pressure for sleep during wakeful, daylight hours.

I believe there is another component that regulates sleep. I call this *automaticity.* People who sleep well usually have absolutely no idea how they do it. Perhaps you have asked them! My point is that the *automatic* nature of this type of 'control' over sleep is crucial to normal, good sleep. Contrast this with insomnia, where the would-be sleeper is often preoccupied by his or her sleep problem and its consequences. I call this the *attention–intention–effort* cycle. This is a process that inhibits the natural, automatic control of sleep, and it leads to insomnia. We will be learning a lot more about this and how to overcome it using CBT methods.

Why do we need to sleep?

Sleep is not an optional extra in life; it is a fundamental requirement. In fact, you could survive for three times as long without food as you could without sleep. Much of what we know about the importance of sleep comes from experiences of people who have taken part in sleep-deprivation experiments. That is, where insufficient sleep, or no sleep, has been taken over successive 24-hour periods. The bottom line is that when people are sleep deprived they are not able to function properly during the day. So, one simple answer to the question 'What is sleep for?' would be that the purpose of sleep is to make sure of good-quality daytime functioning. Let's break that down into three components – physical, mental, and emotional.

We touched earlier on the fact that sleep is required for tissue restoration and for recuperation. During sleep, tired muscles recover and new proteins are synthesized. We also found out that one of the reasons that infants and children need so much sleep is because they are growing ... and because they are expending a lot of energy! Equally important, however, is the requirement of sleep for mental purposes. Indeed, among the most striking effects of loss of sleep are inattention, disorientation, and memory problems. This should not be surprising, because sleep loss causes fatigue, drowsiness, and ultimately an inability to remain awake during the day. If we are to be alert and mentally fit in our everyday lives, we need to sleep well. Finally, sleep is extremely important for our emotional functioning. Psychological well-being depends on sleep, too. When we have not had enough sleep it is likely that there will be emotional consequences! Irritability is a common one, and perhaps feeling overly anxious or excitable. It is as if the brain is trying to compensate for its own sluggishness by making us more aroused. Sometimes, though, people experience a more downbeat mood, like feeling rather 'flat', and even depressed, after a period of poor sleep.

It seems, then, that sleep has its physical, mental and emotional processing components, and where sleep quality is impaired, these processes are not able to do their work so effectively.

2

Normal variations in sleep

Having thought a bit about normal sleep I want now to expand on this theme by explaining how sleep patterns can vary, and yet still be 'normal'. There are three main things to say about normal sleep variation. The first is that sleep varies across the night, and in most people across the week. The second is that sleep varies with age and stage of development. The third is that sleep varies from person to person. Let's take each of these topics in turn.

Sleeping across the night

We have already learned that sleep is complex, yet it is also orderly. I want to give you a little more detail on those ideas by describing what sleep is typically like across the night. Let us look first of all at the middle part of Figure 2.1. This is what we call a *sleep hypnogram.* On the left we find the stages of sleep, and reading from left to right along the bottom we find the time line, which has been set here at a notional duration of 8 hours. This is simply to illustrate what happens over time, rather than to imply that everyone should have 8 hours of sleep!

You can see that in the younger adult, wakefulness quickly gives way to sleep and that there is a rapid progression to deep sleep (Stages 3 and 4). This first episode of deep sleep is the longest and deepest of the whole night. The chart has a series of valleys and peaks, with the valleys representing deeper sleep and the peaks lighter sleep. Sometimes these peaks may touch wakefulness. Broadly speaking, deeper sleep dominates the first half of the night and lighter sleep the second half. You can also see that at the end of each sleep cycle there is a period of REM sleep, and that these REM episodes become more frequent towards morning. This explains why people often feel they have been woken out of a deep sleep if woken up early in the night, but may feel that they were simply dozing if woken up towards morning. Similarly, the chances of remembering dreams are greater if you wake during the second part of the night because there is a greater possibility that you were having an episode of REM sleep during that time.

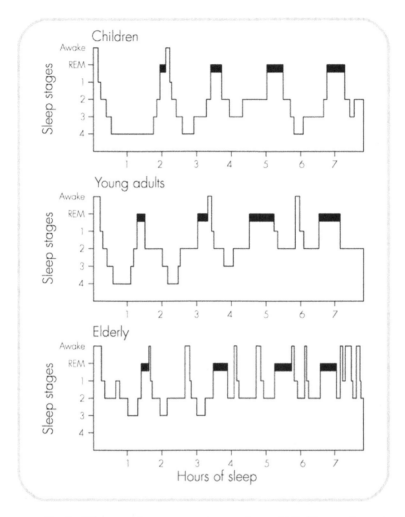

Figure 2.1 Sleep hypnogram in childhood, young adulthood, and later life (Figure 1.4 from Evaluation and Treatment of Insomnia by Anthony Kales and JoyceD. Kales. Copyright© 1984 by Anthony Kales and Joyce D. Kales. Used by permission of Oxford University Press, Inc.)

This pattern is pretty much the same on a night-to-night basis, although it is quite normal to sleep a bit longer at times (for example on weekends) and also to obtain a greater proportion of deep sleep and dreaming sleep on the night after a period of sleep deprivation. For example, if you are up late for a few nights there will be an increased drive towards *recovery sleep,* to repay an element of your sleep debt.

Changes in sleep pattern with age

Everyone knows that our sleep pattern changes across our lifetime. To take an extreme, a newborn baby may sleep 18 hours a day (OK, I know – many do not!), whereas older people may feel fortunate if they can put together a spell of 6 hours' sleep. Figure 2.2 is helpful here because it illustrates developmental aspects of sleep patterns and provides a guide to what might be expected at different ages and stages of life.

Figure 2.2 can be related also to Figure 2.1, which includes a hypnogram of both a child's sleep and an older adult's sleep, to compare with the younger adult we have already considered. Notice that, although the broad distribution of sleep remains similar throughout our lives (for example, we tend to sleep most soundly at the start of our sleep period), maturation and development are associated with some changes in sleep pattern. What I have presented in these illustrations are normal variations in sleep, and this should really lead us to adjust our expectations of sleep according to the age we are at.

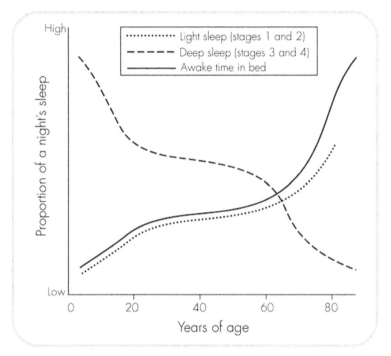

Figure 2.2 Changes in sleep patterns across a lifespan (Reproduced from K.L. Lichstein & S.M. Fischer, 'Insomnia' in M. Hersen & A.S. Bellack, Handbook of Clinical Behavior Therapy with Adults, Plenum Press: New York, 1985. With kind permission of Springer Science and Business Media.)

Few people would deny that children should go to bed progressively later as they grow up, because over time they need less sleep. We regard that as normal, although it is something that everyone has to adjust to. It is equally normal, however, for older adults to sleep less deeply than younger adults, though this may be less widely accepted as a fact of life. There seems to be a natural *fragmentation* of sleep with age. You will see from both Figures 2.1 and 2.2 that the proportion of non-REM sleep that is deep sleep is considerably reduced, and that there is a tendency towards lighter sleep in later life. By comparison, REM sleep is relatively preserved.

We will see when it comes to the treatment section in Part Two, and you begin to consider your own sleep pattern, that it will be important to take into account your individual *expectations* of sleep. In other words, you will want to consider what sleep problem you have in relation to what might be expected of your sleep at this point in your life, and in relation to what might be a reasonable goal for improvement in your sleep.

Taking naps

People often ask me if taking a nap is a good thing or a bad thing. There is no straightforward yes or no answer to that. A number of factors need to be taken into account.

First of all let me be very clear in saying that if you feel *sleepy* during the daytime, rather than just fatigued, you should be prepared to take a nap. If you feel you have a tendency to fall asleep involuntarily, then this can be a risky situation. If you are sleepy while driving or operating machinery, you should stop and take a nap for 15 minutes or so. This type of nap, in these circumstances, followed by two cups of caffeinated coffee, is likely to help you temporarily overcome sleepiness.

However, this is only the case in special circumstances where there is a danger that you will fall asleep. In insomnia, sleepiness of this type is not usual. People more commonly feel tired or fatigued and in need of rest, rather than actually sleepy during the day. As a general rule, therefore, if you are not actually sleepy then my recommendation is that you try to avoid taking naps outside the night-time sleep period. Your goal is to become a good sleeper, and we know that sleeping during the daytime can reduce the body's drive for sleep at night. If having a nap is so much part of your routine that you do not want to give it up, then you should restrict the nap to a single period of no more than 15 minutes, and take your nap no later than the early evening. Let me repeat, however, that if you can avoid taking naps, you should do so.

There is no denying that some people can take naps and still be good sleepers at night, but if you are suffering from insomnia, naps will in all likelihood just add to the problem.

As with sleep itself, there are also normal variations in napping, from person to person and across different cultures. Napping is also more common in older adults than in younger adults, in part due to lowered activity levels, and in part to a weakening of the circadian rhythm which controls sleep and wakefulness. Although I am fairly confident that napping does not in itself *cause* insomnia, I am certain that it does not solve it, either.

Good and poor sleepers

Some people are familiar with the notion of 'good sleep' or 'poor sleep'. You hear individuals describe themselves as 'poor sleepers' and you hear others describing themselves as 'good sleepers'. But it is also very common for people never to have thought about this distinction. Or at least this can be so for the good sleepers! This is consistent with the idea of automaticity that I mentioned earlier – we don't really think about sleep ... until it's a problem.

It is better to think of sleep in *relative* terms, not in absolutes or categories like good and bad. I think this difficulty in differentiating is even clearer when we consider the idea of the 'good night' or the 'bad night'. The truth is that most people have a mixture of these. Admittedly, the good sleeper generally sleeps well, and the quality of that sleep over time is not usually unbroken. However, occasional 'bad nights' do occur. Similarly, the person with insomnia reports sleeping poorly much of the time. I tend to operate on the basis that people with insomnia have at least three 'bad nights' every week, but even they also have nights when their sleep is adequate and refreshes them as it should.

We can see, then, that sleep may be variable for all sleepers, although this variability is much more pronounced in people with insomnia. But why would people who normally sleep soundly have nights when their sleep is disturbed? I think there are three reasons. First, people who normally sleep well do not keep to perfect routines. We live our lives in the real world, and that inevitably involves some variability in how we spend our time. Changes of lifestyle pattern, even temporary ones, have some consequences for sleep. Secondly, the same experiences that contribute to the broken or inadequate sleep of the person with insomnia also affect, from time to time, people who normally sleep well. Take, for instance, stress. Everyone knows what it is like to lie awake at night with your mind racing. But I think there is also a third reason. It may be that the occasional night of poor-quality sleep, or of diminished sleep, has a useful function. Such occasions may provide the sleep homeostat with the opportunity to 'flex its muscles' and to demonstrate that it is working properly by bringing sleep back into line on subsequent nights.

I can sense that some of you reading this are probably quietly seething about my suggestion that people with insomnia have occasional good nights of sleep! Some of you may feel that you have not had a decent night's sleep for years! I respect your sentiments, and my response here would be that I am talking in relative terms. All I am saying is that you are likely to have *some* nights that are better than others. It is unusual for a person with insomnia to have an identical sleep experience every night. You may wish to consider this. Thinking about your sleep in black and white terms is not likely to help you. You need to begin to see the shades of grey.

Others of you may agree that you have a mixture of sleep experiences – and this can be one of the most frustrating things about insomnia. Perhaps you have thought 'Why is it that sometimes I can sleep reasonably well, but I just cannot get myself into a proper pattern?' Never knowing which night is going to give you a reasonable sleep leaves people very frustrated ... and wakeful! The unpredictability of insomnia can be part of its menace, every bit as much as the relentless aspect of being stuck with a chronic problem.

I want to make one other point here. Just as there are people with larger feet or smaller feet, or with larger or smaller appetites, or faster or slower metabolisms, there are people who seem to be better sleepers than others. Similarly, just as there are people who were short for their age in childhood but became tall adults, so there are people who were poor sleepers when they were younger and better sleepers when they were older. Maybe not everyone is going to be the best sleeper. It is worth considering that it may be part of normal variation that some people will be more fortunate than others in the strength of their sleep pattern. That is not to say that your sleep cannot be improved – but just bear in mind that it is a fact of life that not everyone is the same.

What is sleep deprivation?

I have mentioned the term *sleep deprivation* several times already. It certainly sounds punitive! Indeed, throughout history, systematically depriving people of sleep has been used as a form of punishment or torture. We have discovered that the body and the mind can survive much better without food than without sleep, so one can only imagine that deliberately depriving people of sleep would have dramatic effects.

The scientific investigation of the effects of sleep deprivation, however, is relatively recent, and much of this work was done in the 1950s and 1960s. It is interesting that even when sleep deprivation experiments were conducted under controlled laboratory conditions, ethical concerns arose about these experiments because of the risks involved. Nowadays this type of research is seldom undertaken, except in very limited circumstances. Nevertheless, it was through such experiments that we began to understand better the functions of sleep. The specific functions of the different stages of sleep became a bit clearer through studies on selective sleep deprivation. For example, not allowing people to have REM sleep led to disorganization of mental processes such as perception, thinking, learning and memory.

But are people with insomnia sleep deprived? As we have learned, sleep is regulated by the body, and even when this regulation is in some way upset, brain mechanisms will not normally allow us to get into a perilous state of sleep deprivation. We have learned that as we go longer without sleep, so the drive for sleep increases. It is more helpful, therefore, to think in terms of the sleep loss or 'sleep debt' associated with insomnia. Nevertheless, people with insomnia may never quite feel that they have got out of the red and into the black. So insomnia is often associated with a persistent feeling of sleep insufficiency and with daytime impairments to quality of life.

I could sleep anywhere!

You might be wondering why I have put this topic in a section on normal variations in sleep. The reason is that I find there is quite a lot of individual variation in the ability to sleep in different circumstances. Some people can 'sleep on a pinhead', in any situation. There are people who seem to be able to sleep right through a long-haul flight, who adjust quickly to new time zones, who can sleep comfortably in a camp bed ... and so on. And of course there are others who find that they can only sleep under particular circumstances, often only in their own bed, and only if they get to bed by a certain time, and so on. These people sometimes talk about 'catching the moment', or say that they become anxious if they get to the stage where they are 'beyond their sleep'. Most of this I would put down to individual variation – people are different – no more, no less, and in that sense it does not really require any explanation.

What is interesting in insomnia, however, is that sometimes people are actually able to sleep *better* in unfamiliar environments. As mentioned earlier, this might be because they associate their own bed so strongly with lying awake that they have a kind of conditioned response to it and are unable to fall asleep. Another explanation might be that in an unfamiliar environment they really do not expect to be able to sleep and, because they are not too concerned about trying, they become more relaxed and are able to drop off.

Of course, there are people with insomnia who have problems sleeping in any situation.

For some it is simply worse on vacation, or when staying with friends. It is not uncommon in my experience for people to dread, and to avoid, what should be enjoyable times because they worry that their insomnia is going to interfere with their plans. This is yet another example of how intrusive insomnia can be.

Owls and larks

I am sure we all know what an 'Owl' is: someone who has a tendency to be up at night. This is the kind of individual who comes to life late in the evening and into the small hours, often being energetic and alert at times when most of us are beginning to feel really quite sleepy. By way of contrast, the 'Lark' is someone who is at their best in the morning, preferring to be up early and to make the most of the early part of the day. The Owl is not usually good in the morning, and the Lark is not usually good at night.

People who have one or other of these tendencies simply have a stable phase position that is slightly different from the average. Usually people adapt to their body clock tendency, and often quite like it; they make it work for them rather than against them. Sometimes I see this expressed in their choice of occupation. For example, I have seen a number of people who have been radio presenters, doing late-night shows, and it suits them really well because they are the kind of people who thrive on being up late. Its then quite a different matter if they are put on a morning show!

How much sleep do I need?

I am sure we are all familiar with the perils of interpreting 'average' figures. If you are a parent you will be familiar with having checked out your child's height and weight against what are called normative values, or *norms* for short, in order to check that everything is progressing as expected. Although norms give the impression that there is a right answer, more careful consideration helps us recognize that in fact we are usually talking about a *normal range.* To take a different example, that of intelligence, the average IQ may be 100, but this certainly does not mean that most people have an IQ of 100 ... or that they should have. What it does mean is that the normal range of IQ is around 100, so that scores between 90 and 110, or even 80 and 120, would be considered normal.

Table 2.1 provides some information on what is regarded as the normal range of total sleep time at different ages. You can inspect this table and compare for your own age group and see what you think. Of course, even when a value falls outside the normal range, this does not actually mean that there is necessarily something wrong. For example, you might expect that most adult males will be between 5'6" and 6'2" tall, but this does not mean that being only 5'3" represents a problem. Here we have to introduce what is known as the *normal distribution.* That is, outside the middle part of the normal range there is *always* a smaller number of individuals with lower and higher scores. Exactly the same applies to sleep. There are people who are constitutionally particularly *long sleepers* and people who are constitutionally particularly *short sleepers.* Inevitably, these individuals are at the outer margins of the normal distribution, but it does not necessarily mean that their sleep is a problem for them. For example, if a person is a short sleeper, but has no adverse consequences, we would have to suppose that a relatively small amount of sleep is in fact sufficient for that person's needs.

TABLE 2.1: AVERAGE SLEEP REQUIREMENTS AT DIFFERENT AGES

Age range
Newborn
Typical sleep requirement
A newborn baby may sleep up to 18 hours. At first sleep is taken across the 24 hours with no dominant sleep period. By 4–6

months sleep becomes more consolidated at night.

Age range
Young child
Typical sleep requirement
Toddlers sleep up to 12 hours at night and normally also sleep for 1 1/2–2 hours during daytime naps.

Age range
Child
Typical sleep requirement
By the age of 4 years daytime naps will normally have stopped and the child will sleep 10–12 hours at night. This sleep requirement reduces to around 10 hours during the early school years.

Age range
Teenager
Typical sleep requirement
During adolescence sleep duration is normally around 9 hours. There is some variation in when sleep is taken, e.g. it is common for young people to stay up late and sleep on into the morning.

Age range
Young adult
Typical sleep requirement
The young adult typically requires 7 1/2–8 1/2 hours' sleep.

Age range
Adult

Typical sleep requirement

Sleep requirement in terms of total sleep time does not vary greatly during the major part of adulthood. Around 7–8 hours is average.

Age range

Older adult

Typical sleep requirement

In later life sleep is less consolidated at night, with 6–6 1/2 hours being typical. However, there is a tendency once again to 'top-up' with some daytime naps.

Triggers to poor sleep

I want to end this chapter with a brief mention of triggers to poor sleep, because this topic forms a natural bridge to considering insomnia. Everyone has some nights of sleep disturbance, and often there is an identifiable trigger event or situation. For example, people commonly report disruption to their sleep pattern when there is something important on their mind, when they are sleeping in an unfamiliar environment, or when they experience some kind of upsetting life event. Indeed, it seems that any change in life circumstances has the capacity to disrupt our sleep.

What I am describing here then is a normal process, but equally normal is the tendency for one's sleep pattern to recover. That is, poor sleep is a temporary experience for most people. In the usual course of events we might expect that our normal, restful sleep pattern will be restored once the stressor or the life change is past or dealt with. One of the research challenges that we face in the study of insomnia is why it is that some people recover well and resume good sleep patterns while others develop persistent insomnia.

So let us go on now to explore insomnia in greater depth.

3

Poor sleep and insomnia

So what is insomnia?

There are two main diagnostic classification systems that we use internationally to diagnose insomnia. These are, first, the Diagnostic and Statistical Manual of Mental Disorders (DSM), and second, the International Classification of Sleep Disorders (ICSD). These large reference books are what clinicians use to decide if a person has a sleep disturbance, and which type of sleep disorder is present. For our purposes we are most interested in the diagnosis of insomnia, and the separation of insomnia into its various sub-types. Several criteria have to be met for a diagnosis of insomnia.

The characteristics of insomnia

In Table 3.1 I have summarized the main features of insomnia. Insomnia is a *disorder of the initiation or the maintenance of sleep.* That is, a difficulty getting to sleep or a difficulty staying asleep ... or both! Some people experience sleep that is *non-restorative;* that is, they do actually manage to sleep but they feel that their sleep is not satisfactory, not like a 'proper sleep', and they do not feel refreshed afterwards.

To meet the criteria for insomnia the sleep complaint also needs to be present three or more nights per week. In other words, the insomnia has to be a regular feature of the individual's experience, and in this sense has to be typical of their sleep pattern. The next criterion concerns the severity of the sleep disturbance. Here you will see that it needs to take more than 30 minutes to fall asleep (on a minimum of three nights per week) for the individual to have insomnia of the *sleep-onset* (SOL) type. For the *sleep-maintenance* (WASO) type of insomnia, the difficulty needs to include more than 30 minutes of wakefulness during the night. In my clinical practice, people commonly have *both* SOL and WASO difficulties, that is they have at least 1 hour of wakefulness during the night, either at the beginning or during their sleep period. Indeed, many have 2 or 3 hours of wakefulness during the night, most nights.

TABLE 3.1: THE DIAGNOSIS OF INSOMNIA

The complaint
Difficulty getting to sleep or staying asleep; experiencing sleep that is not restorative.

Its frequency
Three or more nights per week.
Its severity
Sleep-onset latency (SOL) or wake time after sleep-onset (WASO) more than 30 minutes.
Its duration
Longer than 6 months.
Its effects
Marked distress; impairment socially and/or occupationally; other important consequences.

Another way that we sometimes look at the severity of insomnia is to consider the individual's sleep efficiency (SE), which I have defined earlier. A cut-off point of SE=85 per cent is commonly used in clinical practice and also in research to define significant sleep disturbance. In other words, on average 15 per cent or more of the time needs to be spent wakeful during the night for there to be a diagnosis of insomnia.

The duration criterion I have given in Table 3.1 is that insomnia must have been a problem for 6 months or longer. The DSM diagnostic system actually requires insomnia to be present for only one month, but my own view is that this is a rather lenient criterion when we are considering *persistent* insomnia. In practice, the majority of people with severe insomnia have had the complaint much longer than that. In my clinical practice it is commonly around 10 to 15 years, as an average, so people usually have no difficulty meeting the duration criterion.

The final criterion in Table 3.1 refers to the effects of the insomnia upon the individual. This is important, because it is often the consequences of insomnia for the person that leads them to seek treatment. It may be that the effects are primarily social. This could be in terms of irritability or other aspects of interpersonal functioning, or it could be that the effects are more upon productivity in everyday life, in which case concentration and alertness may be problematic. Either way there is usually considerable distress associated with the knock-on effects of insomnia. For the person with insomnia, an unsatisfactory night is often followed by an unsatisfactory day. Sound familiar?

Insomnia sub-types

We regard insomnia as *primary insomnia* in the DSM system of classification when the disorder meets all of these criteria and there are no known physical or psychological causes of the sleep disturbance. The ICSD classification uses the term *psychophysiologic insomnia* rather than primary insomnia. This is quite helpful, because the name psychophysiologic insomnia suggests a disorder where there is an interaction of mind, behavior, and physiological responses. This state leads to continuing wakefulness in bed and difficulty getting to sleep or difficulty returning to sleep. As I explained earlier on, this type of insomnia is normally verified by PSG assessment. I suspect many of you reading this book will have this type of insomnia – which is good news, because this type of insomnia responds particularly well to CBT.

As we also found out earlier, there is another type of insomnia the suggested name for which is now *paradoxical insomnia.* In paradoxical insomnia, the paradox is that the individual's experience is of having major problems obtaining sleep (sometimes people say that they don't sleep at all), but tests indicate a normal or near-normal sleep pattern.

So these individuals are in fact sleeping better and more soundly than they think they do. This discrepancy between subjective and objective sleep is fascinating from a researcher's point of view, and highlights that psychological factors are central to insomnia problems. Indeed, most of the insomnia research groups around the world are paying particular attention to psychophysiologic/primary insomnia and to paradoxical insomnia, as both these disorders tend to persist if not treated effectively with CBT and they do not respond particularly well to sleeping pills.

But what about the circumstances where insomnia may have some connection with a health problem? At times of illness, sleep can become disturbed. There may be several reasons for this, and they may interact with one another.

Illness may affect sleep in a direct way, for example where there are respiratory problems, or neurological problems, or during a fever. Alternatively, it may be the pain or discomfort associated with an illness that disturbs sleep at night. Examples here would include arthritis or muscular problems. Similarly, illnesses that affect the immune system, such as cancer, or the cardiovascular system, such as heart disease, can lead to disturbed sleep and to daytime fatigue. These are all examples of *secondary insomnia.* Other examples of secondary insomnia can be drawn from the psychological and psychiatric field, because insomnia can be associated with mental ill health. Anxiety disorders and depression come immediately to mind. If you are stressed, anxious or depressed, it is quite likely that you will sleep poorly.

It is important to differentiate primary/psychophysiologic insomnia from insomnia associated with another disorder, because insomnia should not in these circumstances be considered in total isolation. On the other hand, if you have a physical health problem or a psychological problem, it does not mean that your insomnia cannot be improved using CBT. It's just that you should pay attention to the *association* between the two and discuss this with your doctor. There is increasing evidence that CBT can in fact be helpful even for secondary insomnia. For example, CBT programs for insomnia associated with physical illnesses have been developed by Dr Kenneth Lichstein at the University of Tuscaloosa, Alabama. Similarly, in Glasgow, my research group has been evaluating CBT for insomnia in people who have had various forms of cancer.

There are some people whose insomnia is largely related to the use of sleep medications. Normally this is in individuals who have been long-term users of what we call 'hypnotic drugs'. This is known as *hypnotic-dependent insomnia.* In these circumstances, the taking of sleeping pills has become the primary problem. The individual with this type of insomnia finds it extremely difficult to stop taking sleeping pills, and when they try the insomnia problem magnifies considerably, leading to them going back on the sleeping pills. If you feel this could be you, you should seek assistance and perhaps follow a structured program to gradually taper off and withdraw the medication. The CBT program described in this book may be helpful to you, but you do need to recognize that sleeping pills themselves can cause some insomnia effects. For example, some medications for sleep cause *rebound insomnia* when you cut them down or stop using them. This temporary worsening of the problem can be distressing, and in some cases can last for several weeks. I have provided a separate chapter in Part Three to give you more information about sleeping pills.

In summary, then, insomnia is a persistent disorder involving regular sleep disruption and its associated daytime effects. It may occur on its own, or it may be associated with other disorders or other problems. The CBT program described in Part Two should help you with your insomnia, whatever type it is, but you should certainly seek other advice, too, for insomnia when it is associated with physical or mental health problems or with medications.

Other types of sleep problems

I have now introduced the ICSD and DSM classification systems to you, and hinted that there is a wide range of sleep disorders within these classifications. Some of these disorders have similar symptoms to the insomnias that we have been learning about, so it is important that you check out for sure that your problem is not some other type of sleep disorder. To help you with this I have included in Chapter 6 what I call a 'screening procedure' to help you rule out some of these other types of problems. I have also written a separate chapter (Chapter 11) in Part Three, on recognizing and managing other common sleep disorders.

How common is insomnia?

There have been a lot of studies that address this question, to provide us with estimates about how common sleep problems are in the community at large.

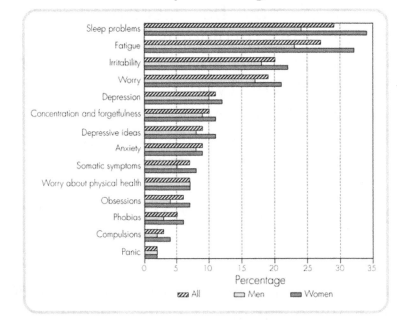

Figure 3.1 Insomnia is a common problem (Reproduced from N. Singleton, R. Bumpstead, M. O'Brien, A. Lee and H. Meltzer Kales, Psychiatric Morbidity among Adults Living in Private Households. The Office for National Statistics, HMSO, 2001. Crown copyright material is reproduced with the permission of the controller of HMSO and the Queen's Printer for Scotland.)

Of course you will be familiar with the argument that statistics can be used to tell us anything! It will be of little surprise to you, therefore, when I tell you that there is quite a wide range of estimates where insomnia is concerned. Much depends on the question that has been asked in a particular survey. For example, if people are asked, 'Do you sometimes have difficulties sleeping?', most will answer yes. Likewise, if people are asked 'Do you think you are a poor sleeper?', up to half the general population will say that they are. Another factor which influences the results of such studies is how many people are approached, and whether or not they are representative of the general population. Needless to say, a poorly conducted study is not going to give us very useful information.

The most reliable of these kinds of studies of insomnia are ones that have included questions related to the diagnostic criteria outlined for you in Table 3.1 (facing). Many such studies have been conducted, and from these we can estimate that around one in ten (10 per cent) of the adult population have persistent problems getting to sleep and/or staying asleep. This figure rises to one in five (20 per cent) of adults over the age of 65. You will see, therefore, that insomnia is a very common problem indeed!

To illustrate this further it is helpful to compare insomnia with some other common problems. In Figure 3.1 I have presented some information from a large study conducted a few years ago in the UK. This was a study investigating a whole range of health symptoms in the general population. The researchers were interested in finding out how common symptoms of depression, anxiety and so on were in order to help plan appropriate services in primary care (community-based general practice). What is very interesting from the results is that symptoms of sleep disturbance and of fatigue were by far the most commonly reported symptoms among UK adults. This was true for adults of all ages, whether male or female, and regardless of the region in which people lived in the UK, or their ethnic background. The graph demonstrates quite clearly the relative importance of sleep disturbance compared with other complaints that people commonly need help with.

So you will see that you are not alone in having insomnia! Far from it. Insomnia is an enormous public health problem, affecting the quality of life of tens of millions of people.

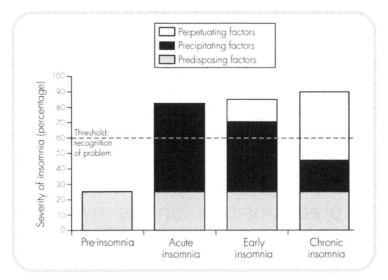

Figure 3.2 Predisposing, precipitating, and perpetuating factors in insomnia (Reproduced from A.J. Spielman and P.B. Glovinsky, 'The Varied Nature of Insomnia' in P.J. Hauri (ed.) Case Studies of Insomnia, Plenum Press: New York, 1991. With kind permission of Springer Science and Business Media.)

From occasional to persistent insomnia

It remains a bit of a mystery why insomnia might develop from being a short-term problem, or an occasional difficulty rearing its head from time to time, to a persistent or chronic problem.

Dr Art Spielman from the City College of New York has proposed a model of insomnia development and persistence that can be useful here. As we can see in Figure 3.2, we may assume that everyone has some degree of *predisposition* to develop insomnia, just as one might presume that we have a level of predisposition to develop any other kind of problem. For one individual that predisposition may be higher, say because of a family history of the problem or having a less well-regulated circadian rhythm, or because of a tendency towards anxiety. As the model suggests, however, predisposition on its own would not normally lead someone to develop insomnia. Dr Spielman proposes rather that insomnia develops, first of all, when *precipitating* or triggering factors reach a certain point. We can think of a wide range of factors that might be relevant here, including temporary changes in our sleep environment, or our home environment, or work-related stresses, illness, acute anxiety, and so on.

However, under normal circumstances we would expect that when those temporary, triggering factors diminish again, a good sleep pattern would be reinstated, and the symptoms of insomnia would decline. The model goes on to suggest, therefore, that *perpetuating* factors are required if an insomnia disorder is going to persist. We can imagine that becoming concerned and anxious about sleep could itself be a powerful perpetuating factor for insomnia. Similarly, in response to such concerns, the person with a developing insomnia problem might disrupt their own sleep patterns further by making behavioral changes to sleep routines.

For example, it is tempting to try to catch up on sleep by going to bed early or sleeping in late, but this might just lead to a drop in sleep efficiency rather than a gain if it means that an even longer time is spent lying awake in bed.

Dr Charles Morin from Université Laval in Québec City has extensively researched the *beliefs* and *attitudes* that people with insomnia develop about their sleep and their sleeplessness. This line of research suggests that the sleep *perspective* of the person with insomnia differs from that of the good sleeper, and that this changed perspective can contribute to persistent insomnia. A common example would be that people with insomnia develop the belief that how they feel during the day is largely a result of how they slept the night before. Therefore, they try to anticipate and to control their sleep at night. This thinking pattern becomes associated with anxious, intrusive thoughts about sleep that are *arousing* and so are counterproductive to sleep itself, and also counterproductive to daytime relaxation.

A model of insomnia development

At my own University of Glasgow Sleep Research Laboratory we have been particularly interested in the process of 'automaticity' described earlier. You will recall that good sleepers are normally quite unaware of how or why their sleep pattern is so well regulated. It just seems to happen ... as it were, automatically. They don't really think much about it. I want to go into a more detailed explanation of automaticity so that you can understand how the *inhibition* of this process could lead to developing insomnia.

Let me start by explaining why it might be that some people go on to develop a persistent insomnia (after a short, acute episode of sleeplessness) whereas others seem to return to their normal sleep patterns. There is a concept in psychology known as *attentional bias,* meaning that our attention is drawn towards objects and events in our environment that are particularly relevant to us. Let me give you a simple example.

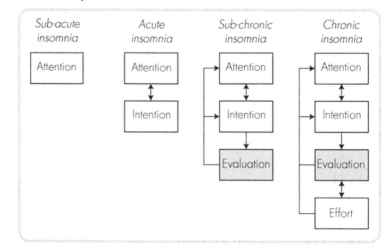

Figure 3.3 A model of insomnia development

One evening last November I realized that one of my headlight bulbs had failed. During the previous winter I had been stopped by the police because of a faulty headlight bulb and had to pay a fine and, of course, pay to get it repaired. As I drove home (not having the opportunity to get the headlight repaired that night), a distance of no more than 2 miles, I counted seven other cars that had one or other of their headlights not working! My attention was only drawn to this because at the time it was a highly relevant stimulus. I am sure that normally, I would not have particularly noticed. This is what I mean by attentional bias.

In relation to insomnia, we might imagine that during a stressful period our attention will be drawn to the source of that stress (e.g. unemployment) and to its immediate consequences (e.g. financial problems). The acute insomnia that might go along with such a stressful episode may not need any special explanation. At this stage, although we may be aware of not sleeping well, we may not pay much attention to sleep, because our attention is taken up elsewhere ... and even if we do think about it we may not think it requires a separate solution! However, there may be a transfer of attention to sleep at some point, perhaps if the insomnia gets worse, or if the original stress starts to go away but sleep does not improve spontaneously. Focusing on insomnia can then leads to further problems with sleeping.

You will see in Figure 3.3 that the development of a sleep-related attentional bias, where none previously existed, may represent the first signs of an insomnia problem ... the beginning of the end of 'automatic' sleep.

This is a relatively new area of research for us, but we have now conducted attentional bias experiments on over 400 people. We have found that people with insomnia do indeed respond more attentively, even to very subtle cues associated with sleep and sleeplessness. One reason we believe that this theory may be important is that studies on attentional bias in other areas of psychology suggest that these vigilant 'response biases' develop in situations where we feel under some kind of *threat.* For example, people who are afraid of dogs will scan their environment and notice more dogs than people who do not have this phobia. I think that the inability to sleep may be fundamentally threatening because of the biological importance of sleep. To be unable to sleep, or to believe that you are unable to sleep, perhaps sparks off a primitive feeling of threat ... of danger. If you have always slept well in the past you may feel very threatened by the idea that something you previously took for granted and never had to do anything about, or even had to think about, has now become a problem.

So let's consider what might happen next. You have become more attentive to your sleep. I suggest that this is followed by an *intentional* process. You did not previously pay much attention to sleep, nor did you have particular sleep intentions ... but *now* it feels as if you need to have a sleep plan. The intentional process is a *planning* process where you begin to think through options and decide on what to do about your developing sleep problem. The intention to sleep, however, is another step along the way to converting what used to be an unconscious, automatic process into a deliberate plan. It is as if you have swapped your car's automatic gearbox for a manual version. You have taken over more of the controls. Consequently, automaticity is inhibited even more ... and, of course, attention is further heightened because you become even more aware of sleep and sleeplessness in your life.

So now both attention and intention are switched on. You are rapidly losing your sleep's automatic pilot. One possibility is that your plan works out well and that your sleep recovers quickly. In this case, automaticity would be reestablished (back on autopilot) and attention and intention would be switched off again. However, if you feel that your sleep is not improving, it is likely that both attentional and intentional processes will now become heightened. I suggest that this *evaluative* process will also directly inhibit the automaticity of sleep, for two reasons. First, scrutinizing sleep performance in this way will focus more (not less) of your attention and intention on it. Second, evaluation introduces an emotional component to the development of insomnia – thinking about success/failure ... anxieties about sleep not recovering ... worry about the consequences of sleeplessness ... concerns about losing control. This last point is significant because the model of good sleep that I am proposing is that good sleep 'control' is automatic ... yet here we have the development of the incorrect and dysfunctional idea that sleep *should be* under deliberate control.

Finally, in Figure 3.3 you will see that I am suggesting that an *effortful* process becomes engaged in persistent insomnia. We already have attention, intention and evaluation switched on. What happens now is that we increasingly try to sleep – we put in a big effort ... we do everything we can ... leave no stone unturned ... we use all the resources we can find ... to *try* to get sleep. This effortful process, I suggest, is also driven by emotion, maybe even desperation. Of course, feedback from the evaluative process is likely to be negative – so attention, intention and evaluation are likely to become heightened further still. Needless to say, sleep effort puts the final nail in the coffin of automaticity. Everything is now anything but automatic. Our work on the development of the

Glasgow Sleep Effort Scale suggests that sleep effort is highly relevant to the experience of insomnia. You will learn more about this scale and how to use it later on.

I believe that it is in the *context* of sleep intention and sleep effort that the person with insomnia is likely to do things that will make it very unlikely for good sleep to be able to return spontaneously. With automaticity damaged, the sleep homeostat and the circadian timer become more vulnerable to our emotions and to our behavior. For example, in my experience people with insomnia often make their problems worse, not better, by changing their sleep patterns over and over. Most commonly, they end up spending too much time in bed in relation to the amount of sleep they are getting, so sleep efficiency plummets, and the experience of conditioned arousal in bed increases. Dysregulation of the homeostat and/or the circadian timer is, ironically, perhaps the consequence of people with insomnia trying too hard to put things right.

In summary, then, I think that being *preoccupied with sleep* may represent the *critical* difference between the good sleeper and the person with psychophysiologic/primary insomnia. I hope that you can see that there is a lot of work going on around the world in an effort to understand why and how insomnia develops.

The doctor's dilemma

It is not uncommon for people with insomnia to feel misunderstood. To a good sleeper there is nothing particularly complicated about getting to sleep, so they may not understand and do not know what to suggest. That's not to say that people do not sympathize. Everyone has experienced occasional bad nights of sleep ... enough to know that it is a horrible experience.

More often than not, however, doctors do not really know what to suggest either. Very often people with insomnia are left with the feeling that they just have to live with it. Sometimes it is suggested that they might be depressed, and on occasions this is correct. Sometimes the insomnia will be defined by what it is *not.* For example, 'I don't think you're depressed', or 'I don't think you've got sleep apnea', as if to say that what you *have* got is *only* something else – something else called 'insomnia' ... which you probably already knew.

I do not mean to be cynical here. I am just reporting what I hear time and time again. But let me provide a corrective to the tone of my comments. I believe that doctors have an extraordinarily difficult task when it comes to trying to give advice about persistent insomnia. Their dilemma is this: they are presented with a distressed person who has a persistent and intrusive complaint, for which they usually have no effective treatment available.

Traditionally, doctors have prescribed medication for insomnia. However, sleeping pills are recommended *only* for short-term insomnia, not persistent insomnia, and their prescription is particularly discouraged in older adults whose bodies are slower to break down the chemical compounds in the drugs. All of the so-called 'hypnotic' drugs are relatively unproven over the longer term, so we do not really know what benefits they have over long-term use. Certainly, many people who take sleeping pills habitually find that they con-tinue to have significant difficulties getting to sleep or staying asleep. The beneficial effects of the medication tend to wear off, requiring either a higher dose or a different drug. In some cases, this can lead to a dependency problem, especially if there are *rebound insomnia* symptoms associated with the medication. Your doctor should be aware of the benefits that can be associated with occasional or very short-term use of various sleeping pills, as well as their limitations and the way they might interact with other medications.

There is really only one other prescription option. That is to prescribe an antidepressant drug, either because there is a suspicion of an underlying depression associated with the insomnia, or because the antidepressant drug happens to have a sedative side-effect when taken at night. The all-too-common practice of prescribing an antidepressant in the absence of depression, however, remains controversial. The most commonly used drugs for this purpose are in a group called the tricyclic antidepressants. However, there are few controlled clinical trials of these drugs for the purpose of treating insomnia, and this is a matter of current debate and concern among sleep medicine specialists internationally.

The treatment with the best evidence of success for persistent insomnia is, of course, cognitive behavioral therapy (CBT). The doctors' problem here is that CBT is often not readily available or accessible to their medical practice. Clinical psychologists, or others trained in CBT methods as applied to insomnia, are needed to treat people with insomnia effectively, and these specialists can be a scarce resource.

Fortunately, there is growing interest in the field that has become known as behavioral sleep medicine. The American Academy of Sleep Medicine and other sleep societies worldwide now have specialist sections for those interested in and certified in behavioral sleep medicine practice. So it is expected that assessment and treatment services for people with insomnia will expand both in association with established sleep centres and sleep laboratories, and in the community at large.

In the meantime, hopefully you will find that the CBT methods laid out in this book will work for you.

4

The consequences of insomnia

Simply having a bad night?

As we know, insomnia is a disorder of getting to sleep, a disorder of staying asleep, or a disorder that involves both of these problems. It is important to start this chapter, therefore, with a consideration of the impact that insomnia has on the *experience* of sleep itself.

It is extremely unpleasant to lie awake at night, unable to sleep and hoping either that sleep will come soon ... or perhaps that morning will come soon. People with insomnia have this negative experience very regularly, and it becomes very demoralizing. Just in the same way as having bad experiences at work, or in a close personal relationship, can lead you to feel low, or helpless, or frustrated, so you can get similar feelings as a result of repeated experiences of not being able to sleep.

If this were a work situation, you might want to change jobs or to retrain. In a personal relationship, you might want to confront the person involved, or avoid them. Usually, when we are stuck in a bad situation we usually want to improve it, to change it, or to get out of it. Similarly, people with insomnia *so much* want things to be different. Have you been caught up in that vicious cycle of sometimes reluctant acceptance, other times fervent efforts to overcome sleeplessness, and then again ... hopelessness when the insomnia just will not go away? Sometimes people say to me that they become so anxious as bedtime approaches that they cannot bear the thought of yet another night of restless wakefulness.

For all these reasons, I find it a bit odd that the clinical diagnostic criteria for insomnia require that there are also daytime consequences to a poor night-time sleep. This is as good as saying, 'So what, you don't sleep at night ... but you get by – right?' Personally, I think it *is* a big deal to sleep so badly, without patients feeling they have to justify their insomnia by demonstrating how tired or miserable they feel 24 hours a day. These days we talk a lot about 'quality of life' – but do we really just mean quality of waking life? Surely we should recognize that life is made up of daytime and night-time, and that satisfaction and fulfilment in both of these areas is important.

Not infrequently, in the exchange of pleasantries when meeting someone I have never met before, I get a further glimpse of how the world at large views the importance of a good night's sleep. Once people find out that I research insomnia problems and their treatment, they often say things like 'I absolutely hate my sleep getting disturbed, it's the worst thing' or 'I couldn't cope if I didn't get my sleep.' Even for good sleepers, having the occasional bad night is pretty much universally a memorable experience! The other response I get, of course, is 'Oh, that's really interesting because I have had this problem sleeping for years...'

Suffice to say that sleep is such a fundamental thing that not being able to sleep is no trivial matter ... for any of us!

Sleepiness and fatigue

Of course it doesn't end there for people with insomnia. Night-time wakefulness is bad enough in itself, but it normally comes with other baggage. The first item that most people mention is sleepiness or fatigue. When you haven't slept well at night you are quite likely to feel not so fresh, not so rested during the day.

I have used both these words, sleepiness and fatigue, not because I think they are synonyms, but in fact because I think it is important to understand the difference between them.

Fatigue can be a numbing, disorienting, even depressed kind of feeling – the 'can't be bothered's, if you like. Fatigue is both a physical and a mental experience. Muscle and mind alike seem to resist our best efforts to engage them when we are fatigued. But you can feel fatigued, or perhaps you prefer the term 'tired' or 'weary' (I think they are about the same thing), without actually being likely to fall asleep.

The tendency actually to fall asleep, particularly to fall asleep involuntarily, is at the extreme end of the spectrum. Fatigue does not mean that we are literally unable to stay awake – that is a different thing. That is sleepiness. People with insomnia are seldom so extremely tired during the day that they cannot help but fall asleep. Excessive sleepiness of this kind is more likely to be the result of sleep deprivation or of a different kind of sleep disorder other than insomnia. Consequently, if patients I see at my clinic tell me that they simply cannot stay awake, that they fall asleep at the drop of a hat even when they don't want to, then I would most likely commence clinical investigations.

Pervasive and enduring weariness – the feeling that 'my get up and go has got up and gone' – now *that* is typical of insomnia.

Problems concentrating

This feeling that everyday tasks are an effort often reveals itself as a problem with concentration. In psychology, we talk in terms of 'information processing'. What we mean is that in order to interact with the world, we need to be able to *perceive* (see, hear, sense) what is going on, and we have to be able to *attend* to what is going on. When we are alert and our mind is sharp, recognizing and paying attention to relevant information comes quite naturally. However, when we are tired, information processing becomes more strained, and involves the brain in more work. This is usually what people mean by concentration – that is, the effort to keep focused on something coupled with the sense that a particular task should not normally take this amount of effort.

People with insomnia often comment that they feel they 'miss things', that they are not quite 'on the ball'. It is as if the brain's information-processing system is not working as efficiently as it should be. Because a fundamental purpose of sleep is to maintain good-quality daytime alertness, it should not surprise us to find that insomnia has this kind of impact. Sometimes people complain that they are more forgetful because of their insomnia. This may be down to the concentration problems – things were not taken in properly in the first instance. Alternatively, it may be harder to remember, that is to retrieve information from the memory store. It is as if their whole mental apparatus has slowed down. This sluggishness in thinking and reasoning is one of the ways that insomnia has consequences for the day ahead.

Becoming irritable and moody

The other main area of complaint associated with the daytime consequences of insomnia is how poor sleep can affect our mood. Have another look at Figure 3.1. There we have it – sleep problems, fatigue, and irritability – the three most common mental health symptoms.

When we become irritable it is often because we are tired, or our attention span is short, or we are finding it an effort to do something that we think should normally be a simple task. So you will see the connection between our mood and our ability to think clearly. In my clinical work, people often tell me that they are easily provoked, or on a short fuse, if they have had insufficient sleep. This is made even worse if they have a busy schedule during the day and feel that they are failing to perform to their usual standards.

A sense of nervous edginess can also accompany insomnia. This may be part of the body's defence mechanisms against tiredness, by making the person rather hyperaroused during the daytime, in order to stay alert. We see this clearly in young children, as they become more tired and bedtime approaches. A very similar phenomenon may occur in insomnia. Indeed, it can show itself not only during the daytime, but also around bedtime.

On becoming depressed

Does insomnia cause depression? Or is insomnia simply a symptom of depression? I honestly think that both are correct.

There is a great deal of scientific evidence now that insomnia is associated with depression, and that it often comes *before* depression. This may be because insomnia gets people down and that, in time, they are at risk of becoming depressed. Another possibility is that insomnia can be an early stage of depression which may or may not ever develop into a depressive disorder. I hope I am not alarming you here, but it is important for you to understand what clinical research tells us about the relationship between sleep and mood. You might be thinking it is bad enough to have insomnia, without becoming depressed as well. Alternatively, it may be that this helps to explain how you have been feeling over a period of time. The good news is that I believe insomnia is treatable, and if it is a risk factor for the development of depression, it is potentially a treatable risk factor.

It is also clear from research, however, that insomnia is a symptom of depression. That is, people who are depressed usually don't sleep well. There are several illness classification systems that we use to diagnose psychiatric/psychological disorders and, in almost every diagnosis, we find that disturbance of sleep pattern, in some shape or form, is to be expected. This simply tells us that sleep is one of life's most fundamental processes and that when other things are knocked out of sorts, it is likely that sleep, too, will become disrupted.

If you are depressed it is important to figure out whether the timing of your sleep problem mirrors the timing of your other depressive symptoms. If it does, then there is a good chance that when the depression lifts or is successfully treated, the insomnia will resolve itself, too.

Coping and everyday life

Thinking about the consequences of insomnia in terms of symptoms (tiredness, mental slowing, irritability, etc.), however, does not tell us the full story. The main impact of insomnia in the daytime is on how it affects *what we are able to do.* People are concerned about their concentration because they feel they are likely to make mistakes at work. They are concerned about their irritability because it affects family life. It is this interference with daytime functioning in personal, social, and work situations that often leads people to seek professional help. Living with the experience of poor sleep at night may have felt barely tolerable, but add to this these intrusive effects upon daytime quality of life, and you have a problem that is hard to ignore.

Consideration of how we cope during the day, however, raises a very important issue. It is not easy to draw a direct line between sleep and daytime performance. For example, we can and do become irritated for other reasons apart from lack of sleep. It may be hard to concentrate if we are taking on too much, or if we are distracted by things around about us, or if we are in too much of a rush. You will find out that analysis of what we call 'attributions' – the connections between cause and effect that we tend to make – is one of the goals of CBT.

Insomnia and its effects on the family

In many respects insomnia is a lonely experience. You may have felt, in the middle of the night, as if you are the only person in the world who is awake! It can also feel lonely in the sense that your bed partner may be a good sleeper; or it may be that you experience loneliness associated with living alone and not having someone to share a bed with.

I find that other people in the family are commonly affected in some way by a patient's insomnia. A common concern of people who have sleepless nights is that they may disturb their partner's sleep, or the sleep of others in the household. So, on top of the anxiety about not sleeping, they have this added worry to deal with. They may lie in bed unsure if they should get up. If they are out of bed, they may be unsure if they will manage to get to sleep if they go back to bed. In this way, there is often a big discrepancy between the sleep pattern of the person with insomnia and others at home – going to bed at different times, falling asleep at different times, waking and rising at different times. This can cause disruption and tension. Indeed, it is very seldom that I see people whose partner also has insomnia. You might think it would be fortunate if insomnia were to be synchronized in this way, because people might then be able to support each other. Then again, that may be the reason why I do not see them at my clinic!

It is clear, then, that insomnia can be disruptive for other people in the family. It can also cause problems in other ways. There may be limited understanding about insomnia, or sympathy towards it, at home. At times insomnia certainly can be a source of relationship strain. Partners who sleep well may find it hard to believe that you have not slept. Because they have been asleep, it may be natural for them to assume that you have been sleeping too. There is also the fact that the family may have to deal with the consequences of your insomnia in terms of your fatigue and mood.

Effects of insomnia on social life and working life

As a general rule, people who have persistent insomnia simply do not feel at their best. Consequently, the other areas that are particularly affected are work and social life.

The work situation can be affected both by concentration difficulties and emotional factors. Things do seem more of an effort after a bad night's sleep. It can be tiring to have to fight off fatigue constantly, and the more we are aware of feeling tired, the more tired we often become. We do not yet have very good research information on how insomnia affects the workplace. However, some recent studies suggest that people with insomnia have more time off work, either through being late in, or through sick leave, than people who sleep well. Insomnia is probably very costly to the economy. There are other costs, too. In clinical practice I sometimes see people pulling back from promotion possibilities, especially those that involve additional responsibility, because they fear that they cannot give their work the attention it deserves. Insomnia causes a loss of potential and a loss of fulfilment that would otherwise be open to these people.

Emotional factors play a part not only in the office or factory, but also in our informal contacts with people in social and leisure settings. Generally, people expect us to behave consistently, and that can be hard if our mood is up and down or if we are on edge through lack of sleep. Sometimes patients tell me that they have cancelled even their most enjoyable commitments and pastimes due to tiredness, and fear of upsetting their friends by appearing distant or temperamental. Everyone is different, of course, but many people with insomnia have social lives that are in some way restricted.

Is insomnia doing me any harm?

Insomnia tends to become a persistent or chronic problem if it is not effectively treated and, like many other chronic disorders, can be harmful in the sense that it poses a threat to quality of life. Although insomnia is the kind of problem that people often say they have 'learned to live with', this is usually said with great reluctance. There is often a feeling of having missed out.

Some authorities on insomnia have tried to suggest that it really ends there, that insomnia is an irksome disorder but not one of any great medical consequence. This is not, however, what the evidence tells us. I have already described how insomnia can be a risk factor for the development of a depressive illness. It can also usher in recurrences of depression in people who have had depression before. There is evidence, too, that physical health problems are more common in people with persistent insomnia, although there is little to support a connection with any specific medical disorder. It may be that insomnia lowers an individual's threshold for ill health, meaning that they may be somewhat more prone to illness. Some studies have even reported lower life expectancy in people with persistent insomnia.

All this goes to show that insomnia is not a trivial problem, and it is well worth trying to overcome.

But I have tried everything already!

How often have I heard that phrase? How often have *you* said it? In my experience people with insomnia are very resourceful. They are not the kind of people who passively accept a problem, or complain about it to others at every opportunity. Rather, they usually go out and try to find solutions. Medications, herbal remedies, behavioral, mental and a whole host of other self-help strategies are out there. People have often tried some, if not all, of them. How often have I heard desperate people say 'You are my last resort!'?

When people have a persistent problem, of any type, it is easy to become dispirited, and it is to your great credit if you are the kind of person who has kept on trying to find a solution. The very fact that you have this book in your hands right now is testimony to the fact that you are determined to overcome your insomnia. Now that you have come to CBT, I hope that this will provide the answer you are looking for.

It is just about time to move on now to practical matters like assessing your sleep, and setting about improving it. But why should CBT offer you an answer when everything else has failed?

There are three possible sources of evidence we can look to, to evaluate the benefits associated with any form of treatment.

The first source is anecdotal evidence, the personal testimony of people who have found something helpful. The logic underlying the power of this type of evidence is 'It worked for me, it might work for you.' This is of course a logical possibility, but there are usually no data to back it up on a large scale. Anecdote, therefore, is not a very reliable source of information because it deals only with possibilities. I am not quibbling with the 'no harm in trying' school of thought, but simply stating that anecdotal evidence should not be considered as concrete proof of the success CBT will have for you.

The second source of evidence comes from marketing. There are many products in the sleep-solutions marketplace (particularly at the pharmacy) that claim to alleviate or cure insomnia. Through being branded as 'health products' they appear to have credibility, and the fact that they are permitted for sale to the general public suggests that they are safe and effective. Again, as with anecdotal evidence, I am not saying that these products do not work, or denying that some people report benefits. What I am saying is that there is not a high level of scientific evidence concerning the likelihood or probability of benefit.

Very few published studies have been conducted on over-the-counter remedies, and those that are available do not reach high scientific standards of evidence. To my knowledge none of these products has been evaluated in a properly conducted clinical trial. Such research work, independent of the interests of the companies concerned, is certainly required. We also need to find out if the improvement in sleep associated with these products is of real clinical importance in treating insomnia. A final point about over-the-counter products is that they tend to be very expensive, even compared to recently developed licensed medications.

The third level of evidence is what we rely on in scientific study to establish the effectiveness of a treatment for any health condition. This is where products and procedures are systematically tested in *randomized controlled trials* (RCTs). It is normal to test first against chance variation over time – that is, the possibility that some people will improve anyway, at random; and secondly, to test against the placebo effect – that is, the possibility that some people will improve simply because they believe a treatment will work. The amount of true benefit associated with a treatment, therefore, is established only when the effects of time and placebo have been carefully excluded. It is on the basis of studies such as this that I am able to recommend CBT as the best treatment for persistent insomnia.

Cognitive behavioral techniques, and component parts of CBT, have been extensively evaluated using RCT methods over the past 25 years. Around 60 trials have been conducted worldwide and have been published in the scientific literature. Data from these trials have also been pooled to determine the overall probability of benefit associated with CBT. The good news is that CBT is regarded, on the basis of this large body of evidence, as the *treatment of choice for persistent insomnia.* Unlike sleeping pills, the benefits are not short-term. Two-thirds to three-quarters of people with persistent insomnia have been found to obtain lasting benefit from CBT.

PART TWO

Overcoming Insomnia and Becoming a Good Sleeper

Introduction to Part Two

This CBT program is based on many years of careful research work, conducted in general medical practice settings. It is a program for people with severe and enduring insomnia, and my aim is to pass on to you a clinically proven and effective treatment. Let me explain what is involved and how the chapters in Part Two of this book will help you to follow the program.

You are best to think of this as if you are attending a course of treatment. Instead of me acting as your therapist, the book, I hope, will do it instead! Certainly I have written it for you with this in mind. Over the next six chapters (Chapters 5 to 10) we are going to work towards overcoming your insomnia. Here is the plan!

Chapter 5 is about assessing your insomnia problem.

In Chapter 6 I am going to review some of the facts about sleep and insomnia that you learned about in Part One of this book, as well as adding some new information.

In Chapter 7 I am going to explain about sleep hygiene and relaxation methods, and how you can put these into practice.

In Chapter 8 we have the big challenge coming up – scheduling a new sleep pattern for you.

In Chapter 9 I want to focus on the 'racing mind'. Does that sound like a familiar problem?

Finally, in Chapter 10, I am going to show you how to put it all together, and keep it all together!

TABLE II.1: THE CBT PROGRAM

Topic
Assessing your insomnia problem
Week
1
Chapter
5
Topic
Understanding sleep and insomnia
Week
2
Chapter
6
Topic
Sleep hygiene and relaxation
Week
3
Chapter
7
Topic
Scheduling your new sleep pattern
Week
4
Chapter
8

Topic
Dealing with a racing mind
Week
5
Chapter
9
Topic
Putting it all together
Week
6
Chapter
10

Going back to that idea of attending a course, I have listed the CBT course program in Table II.1. You will see that I have set it out week by week. That is because I want you to become familiar with each part of the treatment, and to develop the necessary skills as you go along. I will introduce treatment elements a step at a time. This is to give you the chance to understand them and to put them into practice. So here is a warning: this program is not meant as a 'pick-and-mix'. I will be able to help you most if you complete the whole treatment program the way I have laid it out, over the course of 6 weeks. Being realistic, I know that I can't actually stop you jumping ahead – but just remember that my advice is that you go through the program with me, stage by stage, chapter by chapter.

Let me also say that it is not just a matter of reading. The book is more like a manual – a *what* to do, *how* to do it, *when* to do it, kind of book, if you like. Hopefully, you will also become clearer about *why* you are doing what you are doing. Try to give your reading and preparation for CBT some priority time so that you can make the most of the advice I can give you. If you were really attending a CBT course you would be setting aside a couple of hours for that at least. Plus you would have the 'homework' aspect to it, too, because you would be putting into practice what you had learned. You need to follow this same kind of discipline here if you want to get the most benefit from the book. Have a think now about when you can set aside time each week to concentrate on the material you need to cover.

I think of your task as a cycle of reading, understanding, applying and reviewing ... as you go along. It's good to go back over things again and again to make sure that you really understand. As you put things into practice you will understand even better. By reviewing how things are going with your sleep pattern, you will be giving yourself feedback on your success in applying what you have learned and will have the opportunity to check if you are following each part of the CBT program correctly. On the next read-through, perhaps you will pick up on something else. I'm sure you get what I mean – the bottom line is that this course requires quite a bit from you. Keep going round that cycle.

Another practical point – don't just rely on your memory! Get yourself a notebook where you can jot down important points from time to time. I will refer to using your notebook as we go along ... so be prepared.

Having said all this, I don't want you to be too daunted. This is a very practical program using plain English to introduce CBT techniques that have been found to be effective for insomnia.

5

Assessing your insomnia problem (Program Week 1)

Introduction

This is the first week of the CBT program, and we start off with assessment. In CBT, assessment and treatment go hand in hand. You will see as we go through the program that you are often pausing to assess some aspect of your sleep, or some aspect of your behavior or attitude concerning sleep.

The chapter starts by helping you with the important task of gathering your personal sleep history. We need to consider what your sleep pattern has been like over the years, and how, and possibly when, your insomnia developed. We also need to be sure that what we are dealing with is indeed insomnia, and not some other type of sleep disorder. I will introduce you to the Sleep Diary, an invaluable tool in CBT for insomnia, and I will coach you in how to use it. Bit by bit you will be able to form a clear picture of what kind of shape your sleep pattern is in. We will then move on to a consideration of your goals – that is, what you are hoping for as a result of successful treatment. Finally, this chapter concludes with help for assessing your motivational state – your readiness for CBT.

Aim

The purpose of this chapter is *to provide you with the means to assess the nature and severity of your sleep problem and its impact upon your life.*

Your personal sleep history

Those of us who work in clinical practice talk about 'taking a history'. What we mean is finding out as much as we can about a problem, about how it shows itself day to day, and about its development over a period of time. In simple terms, the idea is to obtain an accurate picture. Here, of course, we are concerned with your *personal* sleep history.

Obviously I cannot take your history. What I can do, though, is to provide you with a structure that will help you to discover your own sleep history. You will see there is a format for this in Table 5.1. This is what is called a *semi-structured* approach because it guides you to general areas of content (left column) and to ask yourself 'starter' questions (middle column) at first to focus upon the issues of interest. In the right-hand column I have given you some further questions to answer to go into topics in more detail.

Is now a good time for you to work your way through your sleep history? Now where did you put that notebook? You will find a notebook really helpful throughout the CBT program, because writing things down does help us to think about them and to figure them out. In doing your history you may find you have to check out some information with other people – perhaps a partner can recall important times or dates or events, or a parent or brother or sister may remember further back when you were younger. Your notebook is also going to be helpful when it comes to reminding you of key points in the program, and of the decisions and plans you have made for your sleep. Oh, and before I leave the topic of notebooks, don't get too hung up on being neat and tidy. Your notebook is ... for taking notes. It doesn't need to be a thing of beauty or a work of art. Use your notebook as a working document or a working file – if you really want to have a finished product at the end of the day, you can write that up later from your notes.

You can see in Table 5.1 that the sleep history begins with your sleep pattern, its quality and how it is affecting you. At this stage try to think of these matters fairly generally, because later I will be introducing the use of a Sleep Diary that will help you collect some of this information in a more systematic way. Next in Table 5.1 you will see you are moving on to consider how and when your insomnia developed over the years and how you used to sleep when you were younger. As I mentioned, some of this might need to be discussed with other people who have useful information to share. Moving on again, spend a bit of time considering whether other people in your family have had sleep problems, and whether their problem is like your problem, or different from it. It's important next to take into account your general health and psychological well-being, and how such factors might be associated in some way with poor sleep. Finally in Table 5.1 I have asked you to think through and note down things you have tried before to improve your sleep, for how long you tried them, and how well you think you tried them. This is important in itself to have as a record. It is also important because your past experience will have an effect upon your expectation of any future therapy (including the one in this book!).

Checking out insomnia and other sleep problems

There is one other part of your sleep history that is important, although I have put it separately in another table for you. These are questions that refer to other types of sleep problems (Table 5.2). That is, sleep problems other than insomnia. The CBT methods that I will describe in this book are *only* for the treatment of insomnia, so it is important for you to consider the possibility that you may have a different type of problem instead, or as well. In clinical practice I call this a *screening procedure,* because it is simply a way of identifying possible problems.

Let's start with insomnia itself, so you understand what I mean. Look back to Table 3.1 on the diagnosis of insomnia, because this gives us a way of screening for insomnia itself. Persistent insomnia is usually defined as taking more than 30 minutes to fall asleep, or being awake for more than 30 minutes during the night, on at least 3 nights per week, for at least 6 months. If you check what you have noted down already in your sleep history you can see if you 'screen positive' for persistent insomnia. In other words, your problem is at least at this level of severity. But you should also have a look back to Part One where I described the main types of insomnia that might be helped by CBT. These were psychophysiologic insomnia (sometimes called primary insomnia), paradoxical insomnia, and also insomnia associated with medical or psychological problems (sometimes called secondary insomnia). Although I have included this last type you will see that it also appears in Table 5.2 because you should screen for the possibility that physical or mental health problems need attention in the first instance.

Turning then to Table 5.2, it is important that you consider whether or not you might screen positive for *any other type* of sleep disorder. Just proceed as you did with the first part of the sleep history. The left column lists the different types of sleep disorder, the middle column gives you a starter question, and the right-hand column asks you some follow-up questions. Keep a note of anything relevant in your notebook. To take the example of sleep-related breathing disorder (SBD), you will see that there is first a question about snoring. That is because most people with SBD snore. However, lots of people snore but do not have breathing pauses that affect the quality of their sleep. It is breathing pauses and daytime sleepiness that are particularly important here, because they raise the possibility of a disorder known as obstructive sleep apnea (OSA). The questions on the right would help you to explore these details further.

TABLE 5.1: YOUR PERSONAL SLEEP HISTORY

Content area
Presentation of the sleep problem
Pattern

Starter question

What is the pattern of your sleep on a typical night?

Further questions

How long does it take you to foil asleep?

How often do you wake up?

How long are you awake for during the night?

How much sleep do you get?

How many nights each week are like this?

Content area

Presentation of the sleep problem

Quality

Starter question

How do you feel about the quality of your sleep?

Further questions

Is it refreshing?

Is it enjoyable?

Is it restless?

How would you describe it in your own words?

Content area

Presentation of the sleep problem

Daytime effects

Starter question

How does your night's sleep affect your day?

Further questions

Do you feel tired?

Do you feel sleepy?

Do you have problems concentrating? Do you feel irritable?

What do you think your insomnia does to your day?

When are your worst times of the day?

Content area

Presentation of the sleep problem

Impact on your life

Starter question

How does your insomnia affect your quality of life?

Further questions

What consequences does insomnia have for you?

What are you not able to do because of insomnia?

How would things be different in your life if you overcome your insomnia?

Content area

Presentation of the sleep problem

Development of the sleep problem

Starter question

Do you remember how and when your poor sleep started?

Further questions

What were the events and circumstances then?

What were the important dates and times?

How has your sleep changed over time?

Has anything happened that has mode it worse?

Has anything happened that has mode it better?

Content area
Presentation of the sleep problem
Lifetime history of the sleep problem
Starter question
Did you used to be a good sleeper?
Further questions
How did you sleep as a child?
How did you sleep as a teenager?
How did you sleep as a younger adult?
Were there previous episodes of poor sleep?
Dates and times?
Did these post episodes resolve? If so, how?

Content area
Presentation of the sleep problem
Family history of sleep and sleep problems
Starter question
Do other people in your family have problems sleeping?
Further questions
Do either of your parents have sleep difficulties (now or in the post)?
What about brothers and sisters?
What about the extended family, including grandparents?
Does anyone have problems that are similar to your problems sleeping?
Content area

Presentation of the sleep problem
General health and medical history
Starter question
Have you generally kept in good health?
Further questions
Have you had any major illnesses?
Have any health problems been persistent ones?
Dotes and times?
Have there been any recent changes in your health?
Content area
Presentation of the sleep problem
History of psychological well-being
Starter question
Are you the kind or` person who usually copes well?
Further questions
Have you had any psychological problems?
Any problems with anxiety or depression, or with stress?
Dates and times?
Content area
Presentation of the sleep problem
Current and previous treatments for insomnia
Starter question
Are you taking anything to help you sleep?
Further questions
What (if any) medicines are you taking now to help you sleep?

> *What have you taken in the post?*
> *Dotes and times?*
> *Are you taking anything you have bought over the counter?*
> *What sorts of things have you tried to do yourself to help you sleep?*
> *What have you found that has worked and hasn't worked?*

My suggestion is that you work through this part of the sleep history and, if you think that you may have any of these other sleep problems, then you should read Chapter 12. I have added this chapter to the book specifically to address such issues and to give you advice on what to do. However, if you think that none of these screening questions is relevant to you, you can simply carry on to the next section.

Using a sleep diary

Sometimes insomnia can be difficult to put into numbers. Ask yourself the question 'How long was I awake last night?' It's not just that it is hard to remember exactly. There is quite a challenge in adding up all the bits of time involved. Also, you may not quite think of your sleep in that way. You may reflect more generally on a 'good night' or a 'bad night', depending upon how you feel in the morning.

This is because the *quality* of your sleep is just as important as its *quantity.*

Although it is not an easy task, I believe it is important for you to try to measure *both* your sleep pattern and your sleep quality as best as you can. This is where the Sleep Diary comes in. I have prepared a diary for you that leaves space for seven nights on the one sheet (Figure 5.1). You should photocopy this so that you can use it over and over while you follow the treatment program. You will get better at filling in the diary with practice.

TABLE 5.2: OTHER DISORDERS OF SLEEP

Content area
Screening for sleep disorders other than insomnia
Sleep-related breathing disorder (SBD)
Starter question
Are you a heavy snorer?
Further questions
Do you have interrupted breathing during your sleep?
Does your partner say that you sometimes stop breathing?
Do you wake up gasping for a breath?
Are you excessively sleepy during the day?
Do you fall asleep in the day without wonting to?
Content area

Screening for sleep disorders other than insomnia

Periodic limb movements in sleep (PIMS) and restless legs syndrome (RLS)

Starter question

Do your legs sometimes twitch or jerk or can't keep still?

Further questions

Is it difficult to get to sleep because of muscle jerks?

Do you wake from sleep with sudden jerky movements or feeling the need to move your legs?

Do you have to get out of bed and pace around to get rid of these feelings?

Are you excessively sleepy during the day?

Content area

Screening for sleep disorders other than insomnia

Circadian rhythm sleep disorders – delayed sleep phase syndrome (DSPS)

Starter question

Do you tend to sleep all right but at the 'wrong' time?

Further questions

Can you sleep well enough but only if you stay up very late?

Are you alert and not sleepy until a long while offer normal bedtime?

Are you sound asleep of normal waking time and can sleep on for hours?

Content area
Screening for sleep disorders other than insomnia
Circadian rhythm sleep disorder – advanced sleep phase syndrome (ASPS)
Starter question

_____

_____

_____

Further questions
Can you sleep well enough but only if you go to bed very early?
Are you very sleepy if you try to stay up until normal bedtime?
Do you woke very early, bright and alert and no longer sleepy?
Content area
Screening for sleep disorders other than insomnia
Parasomnias
Starter question
Do you have unusual behaviors associated with your sleep?
Further questions
Do you sleepwalk?
Do you sleeptalk?
Do you have confused behavioral episodes during the night?
Do you have night terrors when you ore very distressed but not properly awake?
Do you grind your teeth at night?

Do you sometimes act out your dreams? Do you have nightmares?

Content area

Screening for sleep disorders other than insomnia

Narcolepsy

Starter question

Do you sometimes just fall asleep without warning?

Further questions

Do you have sudden 'sleep attacks'?

Is it impossible to resist foiling asleep during the day?

Do you have collapses or extreme muscle weakness triggered by emotion?

Do you have hallucinations or odd sensations when you foil asleep or when you wake in the morning?

Do you sometimes feel paralyzed and unable to move when you wake from your sleep?

Your Sleep Diary will help you to see where problems lie for you. For example, is it a difficulty getting to sleep, or a difficulty staying asleep, or is it both? The diary will also help you look at your sleep across the week. You will be able to see any variability in sleep pattern or sleep quality from night to night, and to compare 'good nights' with 'bad nights'. Most importantly of all, the diary will also help you to assess changes in your sleep as you put the CBT program into practice.

Have a good look now at Figure 5.1. You will see that the diary starts by asking you about your wake-up time and your rising time. These are the times when you finally woke up in the morning and when you finally got out of bed. Next you have to think back and note down your bedtime, and also when you put your light out the previous night. Then there are four questions about your sleep pattern – how long it took you to fall asleep, how many times you woke up in the night, how long in total these wakings lasted, and how long you think that you slept altogether. There is a bit of arithmetic involved! But hopefully you can make a reasonable estimate of all of these important dimensions of your sleep.

It is always a good idea to take note of anything that might have affected how you slept. You will see that I have put in questions about any alcohol or sleeping pills you took the night before. The pills section is easy – you can just put in the number you took, or the dosage in milligrams (mg) if you prefer. For alcohol, I suggest you count in common 'units' where one small glass of wine, one standard (single) measure of spirits, and one half-pint or regular bottle of beer=1 unit.

Figure 5.1 Your sleep diary

Week Beginning _____
Measuring the Pattern of Your Sleep
1 What time did you wake up this morning?

Day 1

_____

_____

Day 2

_____

_____

Day 3

_____

_____

Day 4

_____

_____

Day 5

_____

_____

Day 6

_____

_____

Day 7

_____

_____

2 What time did you rise from bed this morning?

Day 1

_____

_____

Day 2

_____

_____

Day 3

_____

_____

Day 4

_____

_____

Day 5

_____

_____

Day 6

_____

_____

Day 7

---

3 What time did you go to bed last night?
Day 1

Day 2

Day 3

Day 4

Day 5

Day 6

Day 7

_____

_____

_____

4 What time did you put the light out?
Day 1

_____

_____

Day 2

_____

_____

Day 3

_____

_____

Day 4

_____

_____

Day 5

_____

_____

Day 6

_____

_____

Day 7

_____

_____

5 How long did it take you to fall asleep?
Day 1

_____

_____

Day 2

_____

_____

Day 3

_____

_____

Day 4

_____

_____

Day 5

_____

_____

Day 6

_____

_____

Day 7

_____

_____

_____

6 How many times did you wake in the night?

Day 1

_____

_____

Day 2

_____

_____

Day 3

_____

_____

Day 4

_____

_____

Day 5

_____

_____

Day 6

_____

_____

Day 7

_____

_____

_____

7 How long were you awake *during* the night?

Day 1

_____

_____

Day 2

_____

_____

Day 3

_____

_____

Day 4

_____

_____

Day 5

_____

_____

Day 6

_____

_____

Day 7

_____

_____

8 How long did you sleep altogether?
Day 1

_____

_____

Day 2

_____

_____

Day 3

_____

_____

Day 4

_____

_____

Day 5

_____

_____

Day 6

_____

_____

Day 7

_____

_____

9 How much alcohol did you have last night?

Day 1

_____

_____

Day 2

_____

_____

Day 3

_____

_____

Day 4

_____

_____

Day 5

_____

_____

Day 6

_____

_____

Day 7

_____

_____

10 How many sleeping pills did you take?
Day 1

_____

_____

Day 2

_____

_____

Day 3

_____

_____

Day 4

_____

_____

Day 5

_____

_____

Day 6

_____

_____

Day 7

Measuring the Quality of Your Sleep

1 How well rested do you feel this morning?

0

1

not at all

2

3

moderately

4

very

2 Was your sleep of good quality?

0

1

not at all

2

3

moderately

4

very

Finally, there are two questions on measuring the quality of your sleep. I have made this into a simple scale so you can just put in a number (0, 1, 2, 3 or 4) to represent how you feel about your sleep now that you have woken up. The higher the score, the better the quality of your sleep. After a while the numbers will begin to mean more to you!

Hopefully the diary is quite simple to understand. If you think it looks a bit complicated, I am sure that once you try it out over a few nights you will soon get the hang of it. I have made a few other suggestions in Box 5.1 (opposite) that will help you to make the best use of your Sleep Diary. Read through these carefully.

So what shape are you in?

Before you even start using the Sleep Diary I would suggest that you have a think about what you expect your diary answers will look like. You might want to take a photocopy of the diary, mark it 'My Diary Estimate' and fill in just one column (any column) to represent what you think your sleep pattern and quality is like on a 'typical' night. You can then go ahead and start recording your sleep day by day using the diary, and compare what you find after one week with your diary estimate. You can also have a think back to your sleep history and what you thought then about your sleep pattern.

Why am I suggesting using a diary? This is because, in my experience, people often learn quite a bit just from keeping a diary. There may be things that confirm your expectations, and also things that are not what you expected at all! All of this is useful information when it comes to planning your new sleep schedule and adopting the right frame of mind to overcome insomnia.

BOX 5.1 SOME TIPS ON COMPLETING YOUR SLEEP DIARY

DO
- complete your diary within 1 hour of rising from bed
- write down times to the nearest 5 to 10 minutes if you can
- double-check your answers

DON'T
- clock-watch during the night
- worry about it! (it is just a record of your sleep)
- make up answers (it's OK to leave it blank if you forget!)

I want you to *keep your diary from now on right through the treatment program.* Let me tell you right now that you will find this a challenge! It is so easy to forget ... and even a couple of minutes set aside to fill it in may seem like too much at the start of a busy day. Nevertheless, it is well worth the effort and it is very important. Have another look at the tips in Box 5.1. I hope they help.

In science, we talk of 'establishing a baseline'. This means that we try to establish what the problem shapes up like over a period of time. We can then be more sure of whether or not we are making a difference through our intervention. Your Sleep Diary is a record of your problem and a record of your progress in overcoming your insomnia using CBT.

So, what shape are you in? I think your Sleep Diary will give a better picture of that than your general estimate. See what you think!

What are your goals?

It is one thing to come to know what a problem shapes up like. It is another to decide what you are looking for as a solution. What are your goals in using this book? What are you trying to achieve through CBT? I want to think this one through carefully with you, because your success in overcoming your insomnia will be partly determined by your goals. This is an important statement, so let me repeat it:

> *Your success in overcoming your insomnia will be partly determined by your goals*

If your goal is to sleep 8 hours every night, then by definition you would be unsuccessful if you achieved only 7 1/2 hours, or if you did achieve 8 hours but only on some nights. It seems to me that when it comes to numbers, you are best to pitch at the most *achievable* figure that is *acceptable* to you. This is one way that the diary comes in handy, because you can find out what shape you are in at the start. As you go along, of course, you can always revise your goals. I think it is better to be encouraged by making improvements towards your (final) goal, through recognizing progress you have made as compared with your baseline. I would advise you to set realistic goals at all times. If you had a handicap of 20 in golf, hoping to play off 10, would you rather be encouraged by achieving an interim goal of 15 or discouraged because you were only half way there?

With sleep, though, as we know, it is not just numbers. What if your goal is 'just to get a decent night's sleep'? I have heard this so often ... and no, it doesn't seem like too much to ask. However, the problem is that it is hard to know how you go about scoring this kind of goal. How do you define 'a decent night's sleep'? How do you know when you have achieved it? I think you need to find a way to make your goal *measurable.* In Table 5.3 I have given you a list of the categories of treatment goal that I commonly see at my clinics. Which of these, or which mixture of these, best describes the situation with your sleep?

TABLE 5.3: DIFFERENT TYPES OF TREATMENT GOAL

Common goals in insomnia patients want to achieve...

More sleep

They say things like...

'I'm simply not getting enough sleep. I hardly sleep at all and that's no good.'

Common goals in insomnia patients want to achieve...

A more satisfying sleep

They say things like...

'I feel my sleep quality is really the problem ... even when I do sleep, I never feel I've slept properly.'

Common goals in insomnia patients want to achieve...

A more restorative sleep

They say things like...

'I want to be able to feel I can cope with the day ... to feel rested and not tired all the time.'

Common goals in insomnia patients want to achieve...

A more reliable sleep

They say things like...

'What sleep pattern? I don't have any pattern, that's the problem.'

Common goals in insomnia patients want to achieve...

> A more normal sleep
> **They say things like...**
> *'I just want to get 7 or 8 hours ... like other people seem to manage.'*

You may feel that your first requirement is for *more sleep.* You feel that you are not getting enough of it. You may wish to fall asleep more quickly, to stay asleep without waking, or just to get a greater amount of sleep. Alternatively you may feel that the sleep that you do get is not of acceptable quality and so you are seeking a *more satisfying sleep.* Here you want your sleep to be a nice sleep, an enjoyable experience. Another possibility is that you are concerned mostly about the consequences of your sleep. You may feel, therefore, that you need a *more restorative sleep* to enable you to function properly in the daytime. On the other hand, if you feel your sleep pattern is out of control, you may be concerned about the inconsistency of your sleep. This is what I mean by talking of the goal of a *more reliable* sleep, a pattern you can rely upon to be OK. Finally, you might think in terms of wanting to have a *normal* sleep. This might be a goal of sleeping in the way that other people seem to sleep, or in the way you yourself were able to sleep in the past.

The message is to know your problem, but also to know your goals. Write down your goals in your notebook now ... but, because your goals in overcoming insomnia need to be considered carefully, I strongly recommend that you are always prepared to come back to these key questions:

- Is my sleep goal *achievable?*
- Is the achievable sleep goal *acceptable?*
- Is my achievable and acceptable sleep goal *measurable?*

Assessing your readiness for change

The final thing I want you to assess before we move on is your *motivation for change.* Don't be offended. It's not that I doubt your commitment to try to improve your sleep. I know that you are likely to have tried loads of things before. In fact, that is one of the reasons I mention motivation. It can be hard to try again after many disappointments, and perhaps you have limited confidence that anything will ever work.

It is particularly important that I ask the question 'are you ready?' with a CBT program, because CBT can be very demanding of you. I tell you, even to keep up with those diaries will at times feel tiresome! You are also going to face some tough decisions about your sleep, and about your beliefs and attitudes concerning your sleep. There will be things to do ... and things to give up.

Then again, changes take time so please be gentle with yourself if you do not find improvements occurring as quickly as you would like. They say that 'old habits die hard' and you will need to coax new habits to develop! Keeping motivated is the key to feeling encouraged and to achieving permanent improvements in your sleep pattern.

The diagram in Figure 5.2 shows us the process of changing a situation. Where do you think you are on this wheel at the moment? First you have to decide whether you are interested in addressing your sleep problem at this particular point in time. If so, are you thinking about starting the course of CBT treatment, or have you already got to the point of making that decision? Perhaps there are some practical obstacles that will delay you if you don't deal with them just now.

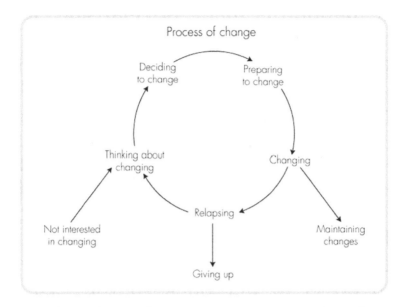

Figure 5.2 Considering your motivational state

If all is set fair to progress, then what are the necessary preparations? So far, that will have involved reading Part One of this book, working on your sleep history, photocopying your Sleep Diary, and so on. If you are on your way to the 'changes' stage then you will have recorded your sleep estimates, you will have started keeping your diary, and you will have carefully thought through and written down your sleep goals.

I want you to come back to this diagram from time to time as you go through the program and ask yourself the question 'Where am I on this wheel at the moment?' Your motivation will come and go; that is to be expected. So do expect it, and recognize it, and then try to correct it. You will see in Figure

5.2 that mention is made of relapsing. *Relapses* are times when you experience a strong feeling of disappointment either with the program, because you hoped it would have worked better or more quickly; or with yourself, because you felt unable to follow a part of the program or you forgot to do it. You may find that your sleep improves but then gets worse (relapses) again. These are all examples of times you may think that there is no point in continuing. Please don't let such relapses discourage you. The best thing to do is to get back to the CBT course and try again.

I want to reassure you that I am telling you this because it is quite normal for the process of sleep change to be an uneven path. Try to think of this as normal and you will find it much easier to deal with. Let me also tell you, though, that you may never have had a better chance of sorting out your sleep problems than this CBT program! Remember it is an evidence-based approach, which means it has worked for many, many others who have seen it through. At the end of the day your goal is to maintain all the changes that you are able to put into practice so that your new, good sleep pattern becomes permanent.

It is now the end of Week 1 of the program ... but before moving on to Week 2, you should have completed one full week of Sleep Diary recordings.

6

Understanding sleep and insomnia (Program Week 2)

Introduction

I can just hear you thinking that we already covered this in Part One of the book. You are correct. Don't worry, I am not going to repeat all that again. However, I make no apology for starting off this first of five treatment chapters with a review of some of this information. Let me tell you why.

> *What we know and what we feel are not necessarily the same thing.*

I would encourage you to read this statement over a few times. It is very important. Let me give you an example. Phobias are interesting problems – we call them 'irrational fears' precisely because the person with a phobia really knows that the thing they fear is likely to be quite safe. Of course, they do not feel that it is safe when they are faced with the situation! Most people who are afraid of spiders, or thunderstorms, know that it is their *fear* that is the problem. They know when they focus on the facts that the spider is unlikely to hurt them, that the thunderstorm is not directed at them ... but what we know (intellectually) and what we feel (emotionally) are not necessarily the same thing.

What has all this got to do with insomnia? Well, in Chapters 1 to 4 you learned a lot about sleep, and about insomnia and its consequences. I would hope that by now you *know* more than you did before you started out. But can I ask you if you *feel* any differently about your sleep or any part of your sleep problem? Do you feel any differently about yourself, as a poor sleeper?

For information to be of any real help to you, it has to change not only the way you think but also the way you feel. In Chapter 5 you began to assess your sleep pattern. Your Sleep Diary will have given you detailed information to consider on how you are sleeping at present. Now you need to weigh up that Sleep Diary information alongside what you have learned from Part One of the book.

This part of the CBT program is partly about encouraging you to have an open mind. Perhaps you need to form a fresh view about some things relating to sleep or insomnia? And to let the facts affect how you feel? I am also counting on the possibility that some of you reading the book will be thinking that you already knew almost everything I have said. But my comment applies to you, too, perhaps even more so. Read the statement above once more. You may already know a lot – my challenge to you is to use this information differently.

Aim

The purpose of this chapter is to remind you about normal sleep and about sleep disorders and their effects, *and to use this information to make a difference to how you think and feel about your insomnia and about yourself.*

Your starting point – a quiz

Let's see how much you remember from Part One. In Box 6.1 I have put together a quiz to test your knowledge. It is to get you thinking.

BOX 6.1 SLEEP QUIZ

1 People need less sleep in later life.
True/False
2 We tend to sleep better as the night goes on.
True/False

3 We should try to make up for all our lost sleep on subsequent nights.
True/False

4 Dreaming a lot is usually a sign of emotional upset.
True/False

5 Sleep is important for our memory.
True/False

6 The more sleep we can get, the better we will feel the next day.
True/False

7 Feeling irritable during the day probably means our sleep quality is poor.
True/False

8 Most adults sleep 7–8 hours at night.
True/False

9 There is really no such thing as 'deep sleep'.
True/False

10 Daytime tiredness may be an important sign of a sleep disorder.
True/False

11 Sleep problems usually pass away quite quickly.
True/False

12 Most people don't cope very well after a bad night's sleep.
True/False

13 Sleeping pills are addictive.
True/False

14 Taking a nap should be avoided if at all possible.
True/False

15 Life changes can trigger insomnia.
True/False

16 Some people seem to be able to do without sleep.
True/False

17 Depression causes insomnia.
True/False

18 I'd be better just giving up because I've tried it all before.
True/False

There are two ways you could do this. One possibility is that you just glance down the items starting at the first question, think to yourself 'True' or 'False', make a decision and then move on to the second question, and so on. That's fine. The other possibility, however, is to take some time to consider each answer. Jot down a few notes in your notebook ... weighing up the pros and cons for both true and false. I think you would get more out of doing it this second way, but it's up to you.

OK – now I will take you through my answers. Some of the statements were a bit tricky because it is not always a straightforward choice!

Quiz answers

1 People need less sleep in later life

The amount we sleep changes throughout our life. The newborn baby might sleep for more than 18 hours, waking only to be fed; most infants and young children sleep from the early evening through to morning, as well as sometimes having naps in the daytime. 'Deep' sleep and 'dreaming' sleep are particularly plentiful in these early years because these types of sleep are associated with physical and mental development. At the opposite end of the age spectrum, older adults who are not using as much energy or discovering as much new information have less 'deep' sleep. Older adults, in fact, tend to sleep less in total than younger adults, and can have more broken sleep, especially in the second half of the night. It is important to recognize that some of our sleep problems, for example 'lighter' sleep as we get older, are just normal changes. Changes like this can sometimes be very hard to accept. In short, the answer to this first point is TRUE.

Now, this first quiz question is probably an example of something you already knew. But let me pose an important challenge to you: have you really adjusted your *expectations* of how much sleep you need as you have grown older? Just because you know in your head that you may need less sleep doesn't mean to say that you have accepted that change and are feeling OK about it.

Perhaps you have never thought of making any conscious decision about adjusting your sleep habits. But things do change. Not everyone still fits into their bridal gown or their wedding suit. Do you remember as a child, when you were gradually allowed to stay up a bit later ... then later still? Those changes in bedtime pattern probably just reflected your sleep requirement at that age and stage of your life. This may be a good time to stop and think if adjustments might be appropriate again. You see, one major problem with insomnia is that we may overcompensate for our sleeplessness by spending longer in bed – to try to catch up on more sleep. The problem is we can then end up with more frustration, simply because we are in bed for too long, compared with our ability to sleep. You may know about this vicious circle already!

2 We tend to sleep better as the night goes on

Don't we just love to get into a deep sleep? It might be nice to think of the night's journey in sleep as one big, deep valley with a flat bottom. That we gradually descend down the slopes from wakefulness into the fertile and expansive plain of deep sleep, and that, with the coming of the morning, we slowly rise up the other side to wakefulness once more. But it's not like that at all. Throughout the night we have different types of sleep. Some of it is 'lighter', some 'deeper', and some is REM sleep when we do most of our dreaming. We cycle through these stages each night. We have several sets of valleys and summits to negotiate on the night's journey. Usually, our deepest sleep is during the first couple of hours of the night, and our lighter sleep is during the second half. So the answer here is undoubtedly FALSE.

But don't take this as bad news! What it means is that nature has organized things in such a way that even if our sleep is short in duration, we get the biggest payback out of the early sleep episodes. These are the most restorative periods, and that is why you can sometimes wake quite refreshed after just a couple of hours of sleep. It is also why you don't need to catch up on all your 'lost' sleep.

3 We should try to make up for all our lost sleep on subsequent nights

This is one of the tricky ones ... but I've just hinted at the answer!

You may remember that I explained about 'sleep debt'? The idea is that during the day we build up a sleep debt that is then repaid at night, allowing us to start ideally with a zero balance at the beginning of the next new day. There might seem to be a danger then for people with insomnia. Not sleeping well might mean that they don't pay off sufficient debt and end up being in long-term arrears! But fortunately this is where the sleep-debt model actually breaks down. We do not need to repay sleep loss on an hour-for-hour basis. The best evidence we have suggests that we need to make up less than one-third of our lost hours. Furthermore, the sleep we get on recovery nights may be deeper and more restorative. I would say, therefore, that the answer to this question is FALSE. We should *not* try to make up for all our lost sleep on subsequent nights. Besides, there is another angle to this question. We should not assume that any time we spend awake in bed is time 'lost' to sleep. In fact, we may not need to sleep all through the time we spend in bed in order to get a satisfactory rest.

The vicious circle that I mentioned in answering Question 1 reminds us that part of the problem with insomnia is that too much time might be spent in bed in the first place.

4 Dreaming a lot is usually a sign of emotional upset

We usually have about six spells of dreaming sleep during the night, although of course some people remember their dreams more than others. Dreams are a normal part of our sleep whether or not we remember them. The answer to this question is certainly FALSE – dreaming is not a sign of emotional upset. It is possible that we dream more when we have a lot on our minds, and there are people who have recurring dreams of a nightmarish quality. Such dreams may have some root in unpleasant experiences or unpleasant memories. In general terms, however, dreaming should be regarded as a healthy experience that is simply a reflection of REM sleep. People may also dream more than usual during withdrawal periods from sleeping pills, and also in the latter part of the night if they have consumed a significant amount of alcohol. These are both temporary factors influencing dreaming sleep.

5 Sleep is important for our memory

Sleep is a time when a lot actually goes on. It is important to realize that sleep is not simply the absence of wakefulness; it is a time when a great deal of different kinds of activity occurs. This activity takes place both in our minds and in our bodies. So although we switch off the lights when we go to bed, we are not switching ourselves off when we fall asleep.

Sleep is necessary for both physical and mental rest. Tired muscles and bodies need to rest in order for our energy sources to recover, and while we sleep our body chemistry works to rebuild itself for the next day. The harder our bodies work, the more we may find we need to sleep. The same is true for our minds. The brain can do with a break, too! But while we mostly stop taking in new information through our senses, our brains are really still on the job. Sleep gives the brain the space and time to sort out information about things that have happened during the day. What we have experienced and learned is processed even though we are not usually conscious of it, and memories are being stored. All this is part of the mystery of the sleep process – we simply can't do without it. There is no doubt that sleep is important for our memory; so the answer to this statement is TRUE.

6 The more sleep we can get the better we will feel the next day

Let me say straight off that the answer to this statement is FALSE. There is no direct relationship between quantity of sleep and well-being. The total amount of sleep that people in the general population obtain follows what is known as a normal distribution. In other words, it is just as normal to be a short sleeper (someone with a short sleep requirement) as it is to be a long sleeper (a person with a longer sleep requirement). The long sleepers don't feel any better than the short sleepers.

Although it may be possible for people who are good sleepers to sleep more than they actually need, there is little evidence that they benefit in the daytime from doing so, except that it is nice to have that choice! There are even some disadvantages associated with oversleeping, because doing so may strengthen what we call *sleep inertia.* This is the experience we have of emerging from sleep into daytime waking with a feeling of struggling to get going. I am sure you have been there. Oversleeping can contribute to sleep inertia rather than feeling refreshed, so the idea that the more you sleep the better you will feel is simply not true. The most important thing is to establish our personal sleep requirement, and to try to obtain that on a regular basis from night to night.

7 Feeling irritable during the day probably means our sleep quality is poor

It is undoubtedly true that irritability can be associated with insomnia, but again this is one of those tricky ones, because there are, after all, many other reasons why we may become irritable during the day.

This is an example of what we call *attribution* or *beliefs.* We know that people who have insomnia will be likely to attribute experiences that they have in the daytime to having slept poorly, but that does not necessarily mean that the insomnia has actually caused these events. I think on balance I would answer this one as FALSE, on the basis that irritability could equally well be associated with frustration at work, difficulty solving a problem, relationship difficulties, and so on. That is not, however, to deny the important relationship between night-time sleep and daytime mood.

I must confess I put this item in the quiz quite deliberately to help you to think through the whole issue of attribution. Think back to the statement 'What we know and what we feel are not necessarily the same thing.' It is important to evaluate your strength of feeling that irritability (or any other daytime symptom, such as tiredness) results directly from your insomnia. More than that, it is important to evaluate your belief in that particular association, against the possibility of other explanations. This process of evaluation will help you to make more accurate attributions. Then you will be in the strongest position to deal more effectively with the most likely causes of how you are feeling. So, for example, you may find that there are stressors at work that need some attention, as well as improvements that need to be made to your sleep pattern.

Going back to the quiz, it would be fairer to say that feeling irritable is possibly related to poor sleep, but that other possible explanations should also be considered.

8 Most adults sleep 7–8 hours at night

How much sleep does a person need? This is probably the most commonly asked question I come across. Unfortunately, there is not just one answer. The amount of sleep we need varies depending on our age, and on what we are doing in our lives. It also varies from person to person. It is important for people to discover their own personal sleep needs, at a particular point in time. That is one of the reasons you are using a Sleep Diary right now.

However, it is in fact TRUE that the average adult sleep is around 7 to 8 hours. If we take all adults from, say, 20 to 80 years and work out the average amount of sleep they have, it will be in the 7- to 8-hour range. We might then say that most adults sleep about this amount because the greatest proportion of people lie close to the average. The problem with averages, though, is that not everyone is the same. Some people can survive on as little as 4 hours of sleep a night, while other people seem to need up to 10 hours. These people are different from the average, different from each other, but not necessarily abnormal.

9 There is really no such thing as 'deep sleep'

The term 'deep sleep' sounds very much like what the general public might say, rather than a scientific description. You might think, therefore, that there is no such thing as deep sleep. However, this is a term that is also used in the research literature on sleep and in the clinical literature on sleep disorders. Deep sleep refers to non-REM sleep Stages 3 and 4, which are characterized by slow-wave EEG patterns. That is, the EEG waves are of high amplitude and low frequency, and are synchronized. These are sometimes called delta waves (see p.10).

The answer to this question, therefore, is FALSE. Deep sleep *does* exist and it is characteristic of our sleep, particularly during the first part of the night. In later life, older adults have much less slow-wave sleep, and so their non-REM sleep contains higher proportions of the lighter Stage 2 sleep. In this sense older adults do not sleep as deeply as younger adults.

10 Daytime tiredness may be an important sign of a sleep disorder

I put this one in to help you consider the differences between tiredness and sleepiness. This is an important distinction to make. Tiredness is almost always present when people feel sleepy, but sleepiness is not always present when people feel tired. I think it is TRUE to say that daytime tiredness may be an important sign of a sleep disorder, but it is important to consider the extent to which you would also be at risk of falling asleep either when given the opportunity, or involuntarily.

There are a number of disorders that involve symptoms of excessive sleepiness, such as narcolepsy and sleep-related breathing disorder. Such disorders will not respond to CBT for insomnia, so it is important to identify them. One way to do this is to consider the tiredness–sleepiness dimension. People with insomnia commonly report feeling tired but do not report feeling that they are going to fall asleep. Quite the opposite: they tend to have difficulty getting to sleep ... even during the day!

11 Sleep problems usually pass away quite quickly

Of course, occasional sleep disturbance is very common. Everyone experiences difficulty getting to sleep or staying asleep at some time in their lives. It is TRUE that these problems usually sort themselves out and end up being short-lived. However, about 10 per cent of adults, that is, 1 in 10 people, experience persistent sleep problems, and this can be as high as 1 in 5 (20 per cent) in people over 65 years of age. There are probably even more people out there who suffer with insomnia but who do not seek help for it.

12 Most people don't cope very well after a bad night's sleep

Many people with sleep problems worry about them. They may worry about how they will cope, about having to take sleeping pills, about whether the insomnia is causing them serious harm, and about whether it will ever go away. Although insomnia is distressing, and can be depressing, people often come to incorrect conclusions about their ability to sleep and the effects that sleeplessness will have.

Thoughts that run through our heads can make the problem much worse. Thinking 'I'm never going to get to sleep tonight' or 'I'll be hopeless at all the things I've got to do tomorrow' is *exaggerated,* and is likely to get us more upset and make sleep even harder to come. Most people actually do manage to cope during the daytime even after a bad night's sleep and you always get at least some sleep. In fact, only a proportion of people with insomnia feel tired after a bad night. You see the body is designed to handle a certain amount of sleeplessness. It can be reassuring to know that even after a lot of lost sleep, it is not necessary to make it all up on other nights.

So, I have put this one down as FALSE. Of course, insomnia can cause problems with concentration, and we can feel tired, edgy and irritable. But we must remember to try to keep our thinking about sleep in proportion. After all, good sleepers get bad-tempered, too. The less you focus your concerns on sleep, the more you will succeed with sleep.

13 Sleeping pills are addictive

Although it may seem surprising, sleeping pills can affect our sleep in a negative way. The pills may help at first, but they often end up giving us problems rather than solving them, once our bodies become more and more used to them. Another thing is that many types of sleeping pills actually change the type of sleep we get, and they are not as good for us as a natural sleep. Because stopping some sleeping pills too quickly can cause severe insomnia, some people find that it is difficult to stop taking them. It is certainly TRUE, then, that some sleeping pills are dependency-forming, both physically and psychologically. You should bear in mind that any type of medication can become a behavioral habit just because we get used to taking them.

14 Taking a nap should be avoided if at all possible

If you absolutely have to take a nap because you are sleepy, then you should not try to prevent yourself from having that sleep. Resisting sleepiness can be dangerous. Then again, however, we might be wondering why you feel so sleepy, if you have insomnia and not any other type of sleep problem. So this also is a difficult question to answer.

If we take it from the perspective that you have insomnia then I would say the answer to the question is TRUE. You should avoid taking a nap if it is at all possible, because napping during the day will reduce your homeostatic drive for sleep at night. A nap of more than around 15 minutes is likely to have some consequence for your ability to sleep at night, whereas short naps have a lesser impact, because they do not reduce the night-time sleep drive to the same extent.

15 Life changes can trigger insomnia

Everyone experiences stresses and strains in their day-to-day lives at home and at work, and there are times when these stresses can be severe. Such times can produce short-term sleep disturbance. However, temporary sleep problems do not always disappear even when problems have passed. This usually happens because our sleep schedule has been upset and poor sleep habits develop, or because we have learned to worry about not sleeping.

Changes in our lives, even positive changes like moving to a new house or switching to a better job, can also affect our sleep pattern. *Any* change is potentially stressful because we have to adapt to it. Some sleep difficulties are initially caused by health problems. Pain, discomfort or illness may upset us both physically and emotionally, and sleep problems may result. Similarly, psychological disorders like depression or anxiety can be associated with sleeplessness, but the insomnia can keep going even when we feel mentally stronger again. My conclusion, then, is that this is TRUE; life changes can trigger insomnia.

Did you identify in your sleep history any life events that might at first have triggered your sleep problem? Take a moment to look back at your notebook and see what you wrote down. Jot down anything else that comes to mind now.

16 Some people seem to be able to do without sleep

I do not know of anyone who has ever been able to do without sleep, so this statement must be FALSE. In a manner of speaking, it may seem that some people hardly need any sleep, but the reality is that everyone does need sleep. Most people can manage to stay up for a night, or maybe two nights, and in that sense go without sleep, but that is a very short-term state of affairs and is not advisable. If we produce a situation where we are objectively sleepy in the daytime, then there is definitely an increased risk of accidents.

17 Depression causes insomnia

Sleep disturbance is a common symptom of a wide range of psychological and other mental disorders, including depression. Indeed, it is unusual to find someone with depression who does not have sleep disturbance. Insomnia, therefore, is so commonly associated with depression that on balance I am going to give the answer TRUE to this one.

However, we know from quite a large number of studies now that insomnia symptoms often occur before other depressive symptoms, and that insomnia is a risk factor for the development of depression. Would it be equally accurate, then, to say that insomnia causes depression? Well, in truth we do not have sufficient evidence to figure out the relationship between the two at this stage, but perhaps how we treat insomnia might prevent or delay depression arising in some individuals. Also we know that treating depression may not necessarily get rid of insomnia symptoms. So even if you are depressed, it would be useful for you to work through this CBT program for insomnia alongside getting treatment for your depression.

18 I'd be better just giving up because I've tried it all before

To be honest, I put this statement in deliberately to be provocative! The answer, of course, is FALSE. You would be better reading on and learning more about how to overcome your insomnia.

Well that's the quiz and those were my answers! How did you do?

Using information to change your mind

The point to it all is that you can use information to 'change your mind'. I want you to spend this next week using the information you have learned, not just in this chapter but throughout the book so far, to challenge your thoughts, beliefs and emotions, and to put insomnia in perspective. You have been feeling out of control where sleep is concerned and now it is time to put you back in the driving seat.

How you view your insomnia is so very important. People often tell me that insomnia has become the biggest thing in their lives. You know that I think insomnia is a 'big thing' too, otherwise I wouldn't have written this book and spent so much time researching insomnia. But

... you absolutely *must* get out of any self-defeating perspective that leaves you feeling powerless and in its grip. You have to step firmly *towards* problem-solving and move decisively *away* from a position of defeat or panic. You need to recognize that although insomnia frustrates and infuriates you, your upset and anger about it are unlikely to drive it away! Instead, we are going to see insomnia as a problem to be solved, a major problem perhaps, but nevertheless one that can be solved.

Evaluating your thoughts

Question: How do you make a start in overcoming insomnia?

Answer: By not letting it get the better of you.

And how do you do that?

By thinking through your thoughts and concerns about sleep and sleeplessness *clearly* and *accurately.*

A number of the statements so far have referred to concerns that people have about their insomnia, and the need to *evaluate* how accurate these thoughts are. Have a look at Table 6.1 on p.110. You will see that I have given some examples of faulty thinking and how it might be corrected. The process is:

1 to record the thought as carefully as you can
2 to consider how thinking this thought makes you feel, and to write that down
3 to reconsider the thought critically – that is, to evaluate it and to write down a new and more accurate version of the thought
4 to consider how thinking this *new* way makes you feel.

Do you get the idea? I want you to start *evaluating* your own thoughts and feelings about sleep and insomnia, as accurately as possible. I have provided a blank copy of this form for you (Table 6.2 on p.111). You should make some photocopies of this and keep them with your notebook. Use these blank forms to write down the main concerns you have right now and to consider if there is another way of putting them that would be more helpful to you. Remember you can use factual information to influence what you think *and* how you feel. Follow the format I have shown you in Table 6.1 by putting your thoughts inside quotation marks ('...') so that you realize that this is the way you are thinking. It takes a bit of getting used to using this approach, but in my experience people with insomnia really benefit from first identifying their typical thoughts, and then evaluating them.

A lot of worry and concern over sleeplessness is based on information and beliefs that are not accurate. Negative or *faulty* beliefs are faulty because they are simply beliefs – that is, they are not necessarily facts. It's your responsibility to check them out – after all, they are your attributions and your beliefs – they belong to you! The good news is that faulty beliefs can be corrected, and attributions can be made more accurate.

Changing them can affect your attitudes to sleep and how you feel. A different mind-set really can help promote sleep!

You will have realized by now that CBT for insomnia involves quite a few paper-and-pencil exercises – your Sleep Diary, your notebook, a quiz ... now thought evaluation forms! I need to tell you there will be more before we are done! Why is this? Is it all really necessary?

Believe me, you will be tempted to skip some of this paper-and-pencil stuff, but please don't. It is important because a person's whole approach to a sleep problem is based on the information they have, how they evaluate that information, and what they then do about it. I don't think you are any different from this general rule. Accurate information about sleep and accurate thinking about sleep and its consequences will adjust your thoughts and feelings about your sleep ... and will begin to modify your sleep pattern.

Dr Charles Morin has written extensively about the relationship between dysfunctional beliefs and attitudes about sleep, and sleeping itself. His research demonstrates that dysfunctional thinking (as in Table 6.1) is common in insomnia, but that changing to a more accurate thinking style is associated with significant improvement in sleep. So I urge you to keep going with your record-keeping in the Sleep Diary and to work hard at these thought-evaluation exercises. I would go so far as to suggest that you keep a fresh copy of the thought-evaluation form in your pocket through the day so that you can write down things as they occur to you. Work away at becoming a more accurate thinker. It will be time well invested in improving your sleep.

TABLE 6.1: EVALUATING YOUR THOUGHTS AND CONCERNS ABOUT INSOMNIA – SOME EXAMPLES

My thoughts about sleep and sleeplessness

'It seems as if I am awake half the night and everyone else is sleeping.'

How this makes me feel

Anxious, annoyed, lonely, jealous

A more accurate version of my thoughts would be

'I probably sleep around 6 hours and have 2 hours awake in bed; that's 75% (three-quarters) not 50%. Also if there are 1 million people living in this city and half of them are adults, maybe 50,000 are having

serious problems. Everyone else is not sleeping!'

How this version makes me feel

Reassured, more optimistic, less angry

My thoughts about sleep and sleeplessness

'I'm never going to get to sleep tonight.'

How this makes me feel

Demoralized, out of control

A more accurate version of my thoughts would be

'Almost certainly I will fall asleep. I always get some sleep. The average in my diary was 6 hours and I never got less than 3-4 hours.'

How this version makes me feel

More accepting, relieved, more relaxed

My thoughts about sleep and sleeplessness

'I'm so tired I just can't concentrate. It's because I slept so badly last night.'

How this makes me feel

Hopeless, preoccupied with sleep, irritable

A more accurate version of my thoughts would be

'My concentration is not just down to my sleep. I've slept worse than I did last night and felt better during the day. Maybe I'm bored, or doing too much at once, or...'

How this version makes me feel

More in control, able to focus

TABLE 6.2: EVALUATING YOUR THOUGHTS AND CONCERNS ABOUT INSOMNIA WORKSHEET

My thoughts about sleep and sleeplessness

_____

_____

_____

How this makes me feel

_____

_____

_____

A more accurate version of my thoughts would be

_____

_____

_____

How this version makes me feel

_____

_____

_____

Remember, you should spend the whole of Week 2 of your CBT program implementing the advice I have given you in this chapter before moving on. Oh, and keep going with the Sleep Diary too!

7

Sleep hygiene and relaxation (Program Week 3)

Introduction

Please remember that I have designed your program to build up over the weeks. These new suggestions are not designed to replace what has gone before! I don't want you to substitute good practices that you have established, because you will get most benefit if you continue to follow previous advice as well as adding in new information each week. So far, then, you should be in the regular practice of evaluating your thoughts and feelings about sleep.

What is *sleep hygiene?* I agree it is a strange term, and not one I particularly like. However, it is increasingly being used, so we are kind of stuck with it now. On the positive side it conveys the idea of the 'sleep basics': what anyone could do to tidy up their sleep preparation, if you like. Sleep hygiene refers to things about your lifestyle and your preparation for bed that might be changed to improve your sleep pattern. Sometimes there may be a simple solution to a sleep problem, such as stopping drinking excessive amounts of coffee. However, for most people it is a case of making the most of all of the good sleep-hygiene practices to make sure that you are better prepared for sleep.

Sleep hygiene can be split into two parts. First, how your lifestyle affects your sleep, and second, how you can plan a bedtime routine that supports good sleep. We will take these two areas in turn, and then go on to consider the very important matter of relaxation.

Aim

The purpose of this chapter is to introduce steps towards *developing a healthy and natural sleep pattern without having to use medication, and to learn how to relax.*

Good lifestyle, good sleep?

The main lifestyle factors known to have an effect on sleep are caffeine, nicotine, alcohol, diet, and exercise. I would like to give you some recommendations about each of these.

Caffeine

Caffeine is a type of drug called a stimulant. This means that it perks you up by having a stimulating effect on your nervous system. Too much caffeine is very good at keeping you awake.

Most people know that caffeine is found in coffee and tea, but many other products also contain caffeine. For example, cocoa, chocolate bars, soft drinks like sodas, and some medicines you can buy at the store for headaches and to help you lose weight. Because caffeine is found in so many different products, I have a suggestion. Have a rummage in your kitchen cupboards, in your refrigerator and in your medicine cabinet. See how many products you can find that have caffeine listed on them as an ingredient. You can use Table 7.1 to keep a note as you go along. I suggest that you make a special point of checking the labels on things you might eat or drink in the evening and before bedtime. Caffeine's effects can last for many hours and it is a good idea not to have any caffeine for 4 to 6 hours before bedtime.

TABLE 7.1: CAFFEINE PRODUCTS THAT YOU USE

Products in the kitchen containing caffeine

_____

_____

Products elsewhere in the house/at work/when dining out containing caffeine

_____

_____

If you would like to cut down on caffeine, or cut out caffeine altogether, you can try switching to caffeine-free drinks such as decaffeinated tea or coffee, herbal tea or caffeine-free cola. Please note that some people who are used to drinking caffeinated beverages on a daily basis experience headaches for the first few days of not drinking them. This is like a withdrawal effect, but it disappears quickly after a couple of days.

Nicotine

Nicotine, which is found in cigarettes and other tobacco products, is also a stimulant drug and has similar effects to caffeine on sleep. Although many people say that they find that smoking is relaxing, the overall effect of nicotine on the body's central nervous system is that of stimulation. What this means is that nicotine will make it harder to fall asleep and harder to stay asleep.

If you smoke, I recommend that you try and cut down in the evening before you go to bed, and that you try not to smoke if you wake up in the middle of the night. You need to consider the possibility that you wake up with a craving for a cigarette and that this has become part of your smoking habit. I know all this is easier said than done, but it could be important.

Alcohol

Alcohol, unlike caffeine and nicotine, is a depressant drug. Normally, depressants should help us sleep, but it has been found that even a moderate amount of alcohol in the evening can actually have a disruptive effect on sleep.

Alcohol may help you to fall into a deep sleep at the beginning of the night. In this sense it is an effective hypnotic drug. However, as the alcohol gets absorbed into your body, mild withdrawal symptoms occur that may be sufficient to wake you up or put you into a lighter form of sleep. Alcohol can also cause you to become dehydrated so you may wake up thirsty in the middle of the night, and need to go to the toilet more often than usual. For people with persistent insomnia, the use of alcohol in an effort to promote sleep is particularly unwise because it can encourage dependence. I recommend that you avoid drinking alcohol from 4 hours before bedtime.

Diet

Hunger can cause wakefulness. That is why a light snack a little before bedtime can help us sleep. On the other hand, going to bed too full can also cause wakefulness. Our bodies are busy digesting the food, and this interferes with sleep.

Yes, some of those old beliefs may be true – milk and other dairy products may help to promote sleep ... if only a very little. Although having a warm milky drink before bed may help you fall off to sleep, it is doubtful whether or not milk helps improve the quality of a person's sleep. I guess what we can say with some certainty in this regard, though, is that it is preferable to caffeinated coffee or tea.

It is probably wise also to avoid snacking if you wake up in the night, as your body may come to expect food at this time. If you do snack at night then you run the risk of continuing to wake up in the middle of the night to satisfy your hunger. A glass of water at the side of the bed is a good idea because a few sips help freshen the mouth and take the edge off your thirst, without causing you to have to run to the bathroom.

Weight changes can also have some effect upon sleep. Too much weight loss over a short time period may lead to short, broken-up sleep. If you are trying to lose weight, I suggest that you aim to lose no more than a pound or two per week, and that you stick to your program of weight reduction until you achieve your target weight. Heavier people are more likely to snore, which can disrupt sleep both for themselves and others ... and losing weight can reduce snoring. In general healthy people are better sleepers, so managing your diet is a good idea.

Exercise

People who are physically fit have a better quality of sleep, so a good way to promote sleep is to get fit by exercising three times a week for 20–30 minutes. The type of exercise you do really depends on what kind of activities you enjoy. It is recommended, however, that in order to get fit and stay fit, you should take up exercise that gets your heart pumping. Walking, swimming, cycling, skating, football, squash, badminton, and aerobics are just a few of the many activities that do this. If you are unsure about exercising, please talk to your doctor before starting an exercise program.

Although being fit is beneficial to sleep, I need to warn you against strenuous exercise before bedtime. Exercise taken late on 'wakes up' the nervous system and can lead to problems falling asleep and problems staying asleep. Even exercise in the evening can have these unwanted effects. So the idea of going out at night to exhaust yourself and then falling into bed is not a good one. If you want to help your night-time sleep, I would say that the best time to take your exercise is in the late afternoon or in the early part of the evening.

Let's have a pause for thought at this point. Do you think that your lifestyle could be improved to help you sleep? Write down any decisions you have made about each of these lifestyle areas in Table 7.2. You can keep coming back to your decisions to see if you have carried them through.

Pre-bedtime routine

It is time now to consider the second part of sleep hygiene – the bedroom itself, and your preparation for going to bed. Noise levels, room temperature, the quality of the air in the bedroom, lighting levels, and the comfort of the mattress and pillows can all influence our sleep.

Noise

You will not be surprised to learn that noise is a common enemy of sleep! Unexpected and sudden noises, if loud enough, will wake most people either from the gentle reverie of the just-about-asleep stage, or even from deep sleep. The cry of a baby, the sound of a telephone ringing, a car horn and, of course, an alarm clock are all examples of these kinds of sounds. However, we know that people can get used to noises after a while, although some folks may be better at this than others. For example, people who live in houses close to railway tracks seem to adapt to the sounds of passing trains. Also, most people get used to noise that is continuous, such as a ticking clock, or even a partner's snoring! Nevertheless, even if people do not actually wake up in response to noises, their sleep may be affected as a result of brief transitions from deeper to lighter forms of sleep.

TABLE 7.2: SLEEP HYGIENE CHANGES IN MY LIFESTYLE
Caffeine
Nicotine
Alcohol

Diet

Exercise

Well, what about you? Try to figure out any noises in your home environment that may be interfering with your sleep, and do what you can about them. Sleeping with earplugs may or may not be the answer for you. If you are troubled by outside noises, wearing earplugs may just cause you to listen in to your own inner sounds, like your breathing. But you could experiment and find out. Probably you will find that distraction techniques, like relaxation exercises, are more helpful rather than getting too preoccupied with something you can't easily change.

Room temperature

Extreme temperatures at either end of the range can affect our sleep. A room that is too hot (more than 24°Cor75°F) can cause us to have restless body movements during sleep, more night-time wakings, and less dreaming sleep. On the other hand, a room that is too cold (less than 12°C or54°F) can make it difficult to get to sleep and can cause more unpleasant and emotional dreams. I would suggest that the ideal room temperature to help promote sleep is likely to be around 18°C (64°F). Why don't you try it out and see? Buy a thermometer and experiment with the climate in your bedroom.

Body temperature

People sometimes like to take a hot bath because they find it helps them to relax. You might think this must be a good thing. However, it may or may not help you to get to sleep. We know, for example, that poor sleepers often report feeling hotter than good sleepers. It is not a good idea to be too hot when you go to bed, so I recommend that you can best prepare your body for bed by taking your bath around one hour before bedtime, rather than immediately before retiring. Make it part of your pre-bed routine (at least some nights).

Air quality

A stuffy room is likely to cause an uncomfortable sleep, while fresh air will promote sleep. Why don't you try opening a window for a bit before going to bed, or adjusting the air-conditioning to give you fresh clean air? The circulation of good-quality air is going to be helpful. Of course you have to bear the seasons in mind. You may not want to leave a window open all night, especially in the winter. See what you can do to adjust that blend of temperature and air control so that it is right for you.

Lighting

Do you remember when I explained how natural light is a major controlling factor in the sleep–wake (circadian) rhythm? We are all familiar with a parent saying that their child can't get to sleep because it is still light outside, or the child waking up earlier in the summer because it is getting light earlier. Natural light, of course, normally penetrates into the bedroom, too – through the window! Don't miss the obvious. Your bedroom at home should not be too bright. A combination of summer nights, or even strong street lighting, and thin curtains should be avoided. I would go as far as to say that your bedroom should be almost completely dark once you have switched off the light. Not totally dark, because that may cause anxiety as well as being rather unnatural. The simplest solution is to cover windows with thick curtains, blinds, or even a blanket during your sleep period. Some people find they can sleep well with a sleep mask on, although not everybody will find these comfortable. If you prefer to have a bit of light, try to keep it very low level, like a small lamp in the hallway with the door very slightly ajar, or a plug-in nightlight of minimal wattage.

Mattress and pillows

There are a lot of personal preferences when it comes to pillows and mattresses, so it is hard for me to give advice that will suit everyone. One thing that does strike me, though, is that we know that people with insomnia sometimes sleep better in an unfamiliar environment. As mentioned earlier, this may be because they don't expect to sleep, so they don't worry about it quite so much. It may be because the triggers to poor sleep – all the associations with nights spent tossing and turning – are left back at home. But another simple possibility is that other beds suit their sleep needs better than their bed at home.

Could any of this apply to you? For example, beds in hotels are often larger and have firmer mattresses than domestic beds. Remember, too, that beds and mattresses of different qualities have differing life spans. A bed can be one of those things where what you pay for is what you get. You can experiment a bit, though. For example, if you have a soft mattress you can make it firmer by placing a board underneath it. But if you can feel the springs, it is certainly time to buy a new one. You may also wish to try switching beds if there are others in your home, to see if you can find the level of comfort you need before purchasing. And salespeople in stores can actually be quite helpful.

There is no real standard for pillows. What people prefer and find most suitable depends a lot on personal taste. But don't make assumptions – be prepared to experiment again. Remember that you don't sleep well – so why are you convinced that you 'need' two pillows? Maybe no pillows would work! Also make sure that you don't have any allergies to the pillow contents, and keep your pillows and pillowslips clean by laundering them regularly. Same goes for your bed linen/duvet. It is also worth considering the amount of bed-covering you need for comfort, and the weight of covering that best suits you.

TABLE 7.3: SLEEP HYGIENE CHANGES IN MY BEDROOM ENVIRONMENT

Noise

_____

_____

Temperature

_____

_____

Air quality

_____

_____

Lighting

_____

_____

Mattress/pillows

_____

_____

Just as you did with lifestyle factors, I would like you now to use Table 7.3 to note down things that you think you need to consider about your bedroom and your sleep.

So here is where we have got to so far with this thing called sleep hygiene. Figure 7.1 will help you to get the bigger picture of lifestyle and bedroom factors that might affect your sleep.

Bedtime wind-down

It is a completely ridiculous idea to expect that you will just fall into bed and fall asleep because you happen to believe it is 'bedtime'. OK, you are going to say that some people can! Well, maybe so. But on the other hand, *you* have got a sleep problem and they don't. And then again, maybe it is more common for people who sleep well to be good at winding down before bedtime.

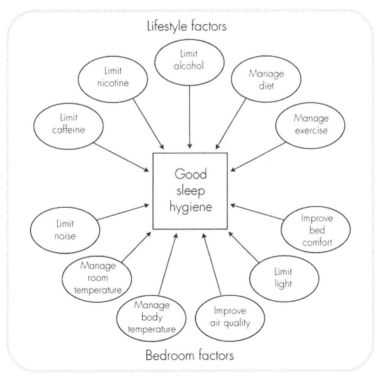

Figure 7.1 Sleep hygiene factors to improve your sleep pattern

I am going to suggest to you that you should develop a *wind-down* routine starting at least 60–90 minutes before bed so that you can start relaxing and preparing for sleep. Your routine should include things like slowing down your work/activity and then stopping it, and having some time to do a number of other things before getting into the immediate pre-bed activities of locking up, brushing your teeth, putting your pyjamas on, setting your alarm clock, and so on. Your routine should be on the one hand carefully planned, but on the other hand should not be rigid or inflexible. I have provided you with a planner (Figure 7.2) that you will need to personalize to suit your own times and activities.

Approximate evening time	Planned schedule
7:45–8:30	Complete work/household activities of primary importance
8:30–10:00	Complete other activities
10:00–11:15	Work/activity completed
	Relaxation time (reading, TV, relaxation exercises, etc.)
11:15	Pre-bed sequence (lock up, change, wash.)
11:30	Retire to bed
	Practice relaxation

Figure 7.2 The bedtime wind-down

Just a few tips, and then it is up to you to consider the detail. It is a good idea to sit down an hour or so before bedtime with a decaffeinated drink and a light snack, perhaps after a warm bath. You could read or watch TV or listen to some relaxing music, or have some pleasant conversation, or indeed a combination of all these things. The important thing is that this period before retiring to bed should help you start unwinding.

Remember that for many people this may be the one period of the day when they have some time for themselves. If this is the case for you, then you can make this time special by doing some things that you like, but with the purpose of relaxing and getting ready to sleep.

Learning to relax

How often have you thought 'If only I could relax, I would be able to sleep'? Well, there has to be truth in that. A relaxed state is certainly a prerequisite for sleep. But can you really learn to relax? I think you can.

I want you to be able to get nice and relaxed in preparation for falling asleep. More than that, in fact, I want you to become a more relaxed person! Fortunately, learning to relax is a general skill, one that can help you in a number of circumstances to take a more relaxed and less anxious approach. Practising a more relaxed approach in the day is helpful in itself, but it is also helpful with both technique and attitude at night. So how do you relax?

The grid in Box 7.1 shows you that there are really two types of *relaxation.* There is the relaxation that we get from *active* pursuits: 'high energy' relaxation, if you like, where we burn up physical and mental stress. Then there is more *passive* relaxation, which is like 'letting go' rather than burning up. I have given you an example of each combination of relaxation approaches in Box 7.1. I suggest that to be a good all-rounder at relaxing you might want to pick up on something that suits you in each of the four quadrants. Easier said than done, I know, but worth a thought or two nonetheless.

BOX 7.1 DIFFERENT TYPES OF RELAXATION

- Working out at the gym
- Doing crossword puzzles
- Gently strolling
- Listening to music

Of course, there are things that are kind of in-between (more or less active, more or less passive), but hopefully you get my point. We all need to have more than one tool in the toolbox. Why don't you get that notebook out and try brainstorming as many examples as you can? Get someone to help if you like. Then hopefully you will be spoiled for choice in the things that you might try. If you don't come up with many options, or if you don't fancy any of them, then perhaps you don't like relaxing! That would be another challenge.

In my experience, people with insomnia often have difficulty with the *passive* approach to relaxation, the letting-go bit. Did you struggle for ideas there? It's so important with sleep that we learn to let it happen and not try to force it. I've decided, therefore, that I should try to give you a way of learning how to relax by letting go, using a technique that I use with my patients in my insomnia CBT clinic. The research evidence is that all relaxation methods have a similar effect, be they autogenic training, meditation, self-hypnosis, or muscular relaxation.

The technique I use is called *progressive relaxation training* and it includes components from other relaxation procedures. Progressive relaxation training includes the tensing and relaxing of the main muscle groups, which lead to decreases in muscle activity, blood pressure, and heart rate. It also includes help with breathing control and imagery (picturing) of relaxation responses.

Here is the text of what I say to my patients when I am going through relaxation training with them. Giving you this is the easiest way I can think of to help you learn the technique. One suggestion is that you read the text out slowly and record it (once you are familiar with it). That would give you a tape that you could listen to, to guide your practice. If you do it properly the exercises should take 12–15 minutes.

These exercises are designed to help you relax. Relaxation is a skill which you can learn. It is just like any other skill, so don't be surprised if you find it takes practice, because that is how we learn skills. So do practice. Practice a couple of times a day, especially as you start to learn.

It is best to practice at a time when you know you won't be disturbed. The exercises will last between 12 and 15 minutes, so you will need at least that length of time set aside. When you do your relaxation exercises in your bed you will be able to listen to the tape there, too. But after a while you will have learned what to do and you will be able to follow the exercises in your own mind.

Settle yourself down. Lie down with your hands and arms by your sides; have your eyes closed. That's good.

We will start by just thinking about your breathing. Your breathing can help you relax; the more deep and relaxed it is, the better you will feel and the more in control you will feel. So begin by taking some slow regular breaths. Do that now. Breathe in fully, fill up your lungs fully; breathe in, hold your breath for a few seconds now, and let go, breathe out ... Do that again, another deep breath, filling your lungs fully when you breathe in, hold it ... and relax, breathe out. Continue in your own time, noticing that each time you breathe in the muscles in your chest tighten up, and as you breathe out there is a sense of letting go. You can think the word 'relax' each time you breathe out. This will remind you that breathing out helps you relax. It will also help you use this word to tell yourself to relax whenever you need to. You will find that your body will begin to respond. Breathing slowly, comfortably, regularly, and deeply; thinking the word 'relax' every time you breathe out; enjoying just lying still and having these moments to relax, concentrating on the exercises.

Now I'd like you to turn your attention to your arms and hands. I'd like you to create some tension in your hands and arms by pressing your fingers into the palms of your hands and making fists. Do that with both hands now. Feel the tension in your hands, feel the tension in your fingers and your wrists, feel the tension in your forearms. Notice what it is like. Keep it going ... and now relax. Let those hands flop. Let them do whatever they want to do; just let them relax. Breathing slowly and deeply, you will find that your fingers will just straighten out and flop, and your hands and arms will feel more relaxed. Allow them to sink into the bed; just allow your arms to be heavy. Breathing slowly and deeply, thinking the word 'relax' each time you breathe out, and finding that your hands and arms just relax more and more and more. Your arms and your hands are so heavy and rested. It's almost as if you couldn't be bothered moving them. Just because you have let go of the energy and tension that was in the muscles there. Breathing slowly and deeply, both your hands, both your arms, heavy and rested. Let go of the energy and tension that was in the muscles there, breathing slowly and deeply. Both your hands, both your arms, heavy and rested and relaxed.

I'd like you to turn your attention now to your neck and shoulders. Again we're going to get your neck and shoulders into a state of relaxation following some tension we're going to introduce. I'd like you to do that by pulling your shoulders up towards your ears. Now, do that; pull your shoulders up towards your ears. Feel the tension across the back of your neck, across the top of your back and in your shoulders. Feel the tension, keep it going not so much that it's sore, but keep it constant. Feel it, and now let go ... relax; go back to breathing slowly and deeply. Let that *tension drain away, let it go. Breathe deeply, and as you do so, notice that the tension, almost like a stream, drains away from your neck, across your shoulders, down the upper part of your arms, down the lower part of your arms and out through your fingertips. Draining out and leaving a sense of warmth and relaxation deep in your muscles. Breathing slowly and deeply and allowing that to take place. Just let the tension go. If it doesn't seem to go, don't force it, it will go itself. Be confident about that. Just breathe slowly and deeply and allow yourself to be relaxed; remembering to think the word 'relax' each time you breathe out. Using that word 'relax' to focus on the sense of relaxation that you get, using the word 'relax' to remind you of the success you are having in relaxing your body.*

I'd like you to concentrate now on your face, and on your jaw, and on your forehead. I'd like you to create some tension in these parts of your body by doing two things together at the same time. These things are to screw up your eyes really tightly and bite your teeth together. Do these things together now. Bite your teeth together; feel the tension in your jaw. Screw up your eyes; feel the tension all around your eyes, in your forehead, in your cheeks, throughout your face, wherever there is tension. Now keep it going ... and relax; breathing in through your nose and out through your mouth, slowly and deeply. Notice how your forehead smoothes out and then your eyelids and your cheeks. Allow your jaw to hang slightly open. Allow your whole head to feel heavy and to sink into the pillow; breathing slowly and deeply. Allow there to be a spread of relaxation across the surface of your face and into all those muscles in your face. Allow your eyelids to feel heavy and comfortable, your jaw and your whole head; breathing slowly and deeply, enjoying the relaxation which you feel in your body. Relax each time you breathe out. Relax just that little bit more each time you breathe out.

Concentrating now on your legs and feet, I want you to create some tension here by doing two things at the same time; and these things are to press the backs of your legs downwards and to pull your toes back towards your head. Do these things together now. Create the tension in your legs, press the backs of your legs downwards and pull your toes back towards your head. Feel the tension in your feet, in your toes, in your ankles, in the muscles in your legs. Feel what it is like. Don't overdo it; just notice what it is like ... and relax. Breathing slowly and deeply once more; just allow your feet to flop any old way. Allow the muscles to give up their energy, give up their tension. Let it go, breathing slowly and deeply. Notice how your feet just want to flop to the side. Notice how your legs feel heavy as if you couldn't be bothered moving them. Heavy and comfortable and rested and relaxed. Just that little bit more relaxed each time you breathe out.

Be thinking about your whole body now; supported by the bed, sinking into it, but supported by it. You've let go the tension throughout your body. Your body feels rested, comfortable. Enjoy each deep breath you take. Just use these few moments now to think about any part of your body that doesn't feel quite so rested and allow the tension to go. It will go. Breathe slowly and deeply; thinking the word 'relax' each time you breathe out. Just let any remaining tension drain away; from your hands, your arms, your neck and your back. Heavy and rested, comfortable and relaxed. From your face and your eyes, from your forehead; letting the muscles give up their energy. Like a stream of relaxation flowing over your whole body. Let your legs and feet feel relaxed; sinking into the bed. Breathing slowly and deeply.

In a few moments, the exercises will be finished; but you can continue to relax. You may wish to repeat some of the exercises yourself and that is fine. You may wish to enjoy just continuing as you are. It's up to you, but continue to relax.

So, in concluding this section, let's try to bring this together. Your bedtime wind-down and pre-bed routine should encourage you to switch off from the day and to relax in preparation for sleep. The progressive relaxation training is there to help you relax even more. Here is what I mean, summarized in Box 7.2.

BOX 7.2 A RELAXATION SUMMARY

Your relaxation program

Here are the steps you should follow for your relaxation program:

1 Wind down during the second half of the night.

2 Slow down or stop doing work/activity 90 minutes before bed.

3 Practice the relaxation routine while in bed:

• Concentrate on your breathing

• Tense and relax your muscles and breathe slowly and deeply

• Take exercises slowly – do not overtense your muscles

4 Practise, practise, practise.

How does the good sleeper do it?

It must be a difficult thing to be a good sleeper, or so you would think! All this sleep hygiene, pre-bed routine, relaxation. Then there is evaluating your thoughts and beliefs and making accurate appraisals of them; the things we were learning about in the previous chapter. Then there is still more to come in the next few chapters – sleep scheduling, dealing with a racing mind, and so on!

How on earth do good sleepers do it? How do they fit all this in? But then there is a special secret. Good sleepers are good sleepers precisely because what they do is second nature to them. They just **don't** really think about it. Maybe they are not even the best at following good routines, maybe some of them have poor sleep hygiene practices! My point is that the good sleeper is different from you because whatever they do is not done deliberately or anxiously to influence sleep. They are not preoccupied about sleep, and so they sleep. And if they don't sleep so well ... because they are not preoccupied about sleep, they tend not to get too concerned about it, so it sorts itself out.

In my experience good sleepers are not students of sleep. What they have is a set of behaviors, attitudes, and emotions about sleep that work. Their sleep-related behavior, the attitudes they have about sleep, and how they feel about sleep and about themselves as sleepers, simply supports sleep coming automatically and naturally. Nothing more, nothing less. 'So laid back as to be just about horizontal' is how the saying goes to describe someone who has a carefree approach. When it comes to sleep and the good sleeper, the saying, almost literally has a ring of truth about it.

I want to help you to overcome insomnia *and* to become a good sleeper. The bottom line is that the instructions and techniques I am giving you in this book provide only part of the recipe. You must learn to mix in the mind-set of the good sleeper. You are going to have to change to achieve that.

Figure 7.3 The thin line between commitment and unproductive effort

Commitment
Being motivated
Unproductive Effort
Trying too hard
Commitment
Following advice
Unproductive Effort
Getting more preoccupied
Commitment
Sticking to the program
Unproductive Effort

Forcing sleep
Commitment
Returning to the program
Unproductive Effort
Trying to win
Commitment
Refusing to give up
Unproductive Effort
Getting desperate

Saving on effort?

I am going to draw a thin line for you in Figure 7.3. Here's the challenge: on the one side of the line I need you to be 100 per cent committed to putting into practice all the advice I can give you. On the other side, I want you to *stop trying so hard!* Motivation and commitment to the program are good; effort and preoccupation are bad.

I know better than most that you feel you are the victim of an under-recognized and poorly understood disorder that ruins enjoyment, not just of your sleep but of other parts of your life, too. I know that you want to beat it, and that you feel you have tried everything. I know that you want to try again ... but I *also* know that a steady, calm, assured approach to doing things is the way to go.

I need you to focus your determination on the left side of the line. Stay focused, follow the program, don't give up on yourself. If you forget or have a setback, pick it up again. If you cross the line, believe me you won't improve or stay improved for long. If you focus your efforts too much upon *trying* to sleep, *trying* to defeat insomnia, you may well feel up for the fight but you will have the level of arousal to go with the battle! Remember, the good sleeper is no conquering hero. You have to stop trying to drive insomnia from your bedroom door and to start permitting sleep to come to you in its own time. This is a theme that you will become familiar with as we carry on through the program. This is what I mean by relaxation.

Monitoring your sleep

Just before we move on to the next chapter and so the next session of the program, just a further reminder to use your Sleep Diary to assess your sleep pattern. I suggest that you keep that going throughout the CBT program. If you've done this so far, well done. If not, it doesn't mean you're a bad person! But I would encourage you to pick it up again and try to keep a note of your sleep pattern and sleep quality each morning when you get up. It will help you track your progress. Also remember to work on all the material in this chapter for a full week before moving on to the next section.

8

Scheduling a new sleep pattern(Program Week 4)

Introduction

Here we go, the new you coming up!

There is a lot to cover this week. What's more, most of the people with insomnia that I have seen find this part the most challenging of all. We are literally going to rebuild your sleep pattern. That means changes – so be prepared.

What I should also tell you, though, is that all of the senior figures in insomnia research agree that this sleep-scheduling component of CBT is the most important one. Incorporated into what I call *sleep scheduling* are procedures known in the insomnia world as *stimulus control* and *sleep restriction.*

Dr Richard Bootzin of the University of Arizona first developed stimulus-control procedures for insomnia more than 30 years ago, and Dr Art Spielman from the City College of New York added sleep-restriction guidelines during the 1980s. These are now the most effective components of CBT for insomnia. The American Academy of Sleep Medicine review groups that I have served on have recommended that sleep scheduling should be included at the heart of *every* CBT approach to insomnia.

You should not take this to mean that you might as well forget all of the advice in the other chapters. But it does mean that I want you to be *particularly* committed to following sleep scheduling through as best as you possibly can.

Aim

The purpose of this chapter is to *reshape your sleep so that it meets your individual needs and develops into a strong pattern that will last.*

Strengthening the connection between bed and sleep

Here is the starting point for sleep scheduling. What is the current connection between your bed and your sleep? That is probably a hard question, so let's start with an easier one. What is the connection between bed and sleep for the good sleeper? The good sleeper thinks of 'bed' and immediately thinks 'sleep'. Bed means sleep. You go to bed – you fall asleep. Bed is a place for ... sleeping.

So back to you. What is the connection between bed and sleep in your experience? Well, I suppose it could be a number of things, but I could hazard a few guesses. You think of 'bed' and you think 'groan' or 'maybe tonight I will get some sleep.' You might even have a kind of phobia about going to bed. Bed means for you lying awake tossing and turning. Thinking about going to bed makes you anxious. Bed means ... a long shift till morning comes. You go to bed – you lie awake, you try to fill in the time somehow. Bed is a place ... for sleeping, yes ... except you don't!

The simple point is that sleep will come more quickly and it will be easier for you to remain asleep if your mind and your body can make a *sleep response* to an important *cue:* your bed. That is how it is for the good sleeper – cue bed, cue sleep! That is where you want to be, I'm sure.

If you always sleep in your bed and if you only use your bed to sleep in, you can, even now, build a strong link between your bed and sleep. This connection will lead your bed to again becoming a cue for sleep, and so help to improve your sleep pattern. There are a number of things I can suggest that will help to make a strong connection between sleep and the bed.

Bedtime activities

First, it is important not to use your bed for *anything except sleep.* This means that activities like watching TV, reading, eating, and talking on the phone are out! When you go to your bed, you should put the light out straight away and put your head down intending to sleep. Sexual activity is the only exception to this rule; it usually helps us sleep afterwards!

I know that lots of people read in bed. And I know it doesn't directly cause insomnia if you read in bed, or speak on the phone. Sure, there are loads of people who read in bed without any problem. For you, however, it is very important that in rebuilding your sleep pattern you get into the way of *falling asleep very rapidly* after you get into bed. I want you to develop a quick bed/sleep response.

You can always read somewhere else, but from now on your bed is for sleeping.

The quarter-of-an-hour rule

Of course, there will be nights when you put your head down and sleep will not come quickly. What I recommend here is that if sleep does not come within 15 minutes, you should get out of bed and go into another room. I know that, just like being awake when it seems like everyone else is sleeping, getting out of bed when you want to sleep is going to be very hard. It may be hard because you feel cozy and don't want to leave the warmth of the bed. It may be hard to know what to get up and do. But there are things you can do to make getting out of bed easier – you could leave the heating on and a table lamp on in your living room. You could prepare a warm milky drink or a decaffeinated drink before you go to bed – because you *will* be awake for more than 15 minutes. You could read or listen to music, or do something else that is relaxing while you are up.

Again I want you to realize the importance of the bed/sleep link. By getting up from bed you keep wakeful time associated with a wakeful environment in the house. Importantly, you also get out of that habit of lying in bed and getting frustrated. If you are not sleeping, you are not sleeping. It is as simple as that. Get up and stop trying to sleep. Sleep will come when it is ready.

Let me say a word, though, about this 15-minute cut-off for lying in bed. First, you don't need to wait as long as that if you don't want to. If you don't feel sleepy it's OK to get up sooner. Second, I don't want you to count down the clock! That is why I call this the *quarter-of-an-hour rule.* This is meant to give you the idea of an *estimate* of the time after which you should be getting up. Good sleepers fall asleep easily within a quarter-hour of putting the light out, so if it's good enough for them, it's good enough for you too.

You should also follow this quarter-of-an-hour rule if you wake up in the middle of the night and cannot fall asleep again. In other words, if you follow this rule you should no longer lie awake in bed for any longer than 15 minutes. This too means that your bed/sleep connection is going to get stronger. Don't be surprised or dismayed if you are up and down quite a few times at first when you follow this rule – it is in a good cause.

Feeling sleepy

It is important that you only go to bed when you feel sleepy enough to get to sleep quickly. If you are lying awake in your bed, you are breaking down the connection between bed and sleep, and you are building up a lot of frustration. So try and stay up until you feel *sleepy-tired.* That way you will be more likely to get to sleep quickly, and less likely to lie awake thinking about not sleeping.

How do you know when you are sleepy-tired? The usual signs are things like itchy eyes, lack of energy, aching muscles, yawning and a tendency to 'nod off'. It is important that you spot the difference between tiredness and sleepiness. Tiredness does not mean that sleep is inevitable, whereas sleepiness is a signal from our bodies that it is time for our night's sleep. We might feel tired but not be ready to sleep, so work on this a bit and see if you can identify clear signs of sleepiness that are typical for you.

The same point about feeling sleepy applies if you are up during the night, putting the quarter-of-an-hour rule into practice. After a while of being up, you should go back to bed *when you feel sleepy again,* but not before. If you still cannot sleep when you go back to bed, you will need to get out of bed yet again!

Avoiding napping

Another thing to do to strengthen the connection between night-time sleep and your bed is to avoid napping during the day – or in the evening. I want to emphasize the importance of remembering that bed is for sleep and night is for sleep. *Daytime is for wakefulness.* This is a fundamental principle. If your sleep seeps into the daytime it is likely that being awake will seep into your night, and this will only make your insomnia worse. Stopping naps if you are in the habit of taking them will not only better prepare you for a continuous, longer sleep at night but will strengthen the connection between your bed and sleep. Sleeping in a chair or on a sofa in another room weakens that important link.

If you feel that you absolutely must have a nap, or if you fall asleep without wanting to, then you have to make sure that you don't have another type of sleep problem that is associated with excessive daytime sleepiness. I covered this in some detail in the assessment chapter (Chapter 5) and there is more information to come in Part Three. The message is, only nap if you absolutely must, for no more than 10–15 minutes – and if you must, just be sure that you don't have another type of sleep disorder.

Summary of the bed/sleep connection

I know that I am hitting you hard with a lot of rules right now, so let's just take stock for a moment.

This is all about strengthening the bed/sleep connection so that it gets to be as it is for the good sleeper. In Table 8.1 I have left space for you to write down any decisions that you face concerning each element of the bed/sleep connection. Take some time to think through *how* you are going to apply each of these rules.

Try not to kid yourself that you will 'just do it' – you won't! This part of the CBT program is very challenging, so you need to consider carefully how you are going to achieve success in putting this aspect of your new sleep schedule into practice.

How much sleep do I need?

How much sleep do you *need?* The amount of sleep that you need may well be different from the amount of sleep that you want.

TABLE 8.1: STRENGTHENING THE BED/SLEEP CONNECTION

Decision I have made about **bedtime activities**

_____

_____

Decision I have made about **the quarter-of-an-hour rule**

_____

_____

Decision I have made about **feeling sleepy**

_____

_____

Decision I have made about **avoiding napping**

_____

_____

_____

Everyone's sleep needs differ, so there is not a single answer to the question. For example, you might have a shorter sleep requirement than some other people. Although you might prefer to have brown eyes instead of blue, or to be taller or shorter in height, you will know that these are things you can't change. Similarly, your sleep pattern will work best for you when you accept you have to work within natural boundaries.

What is more, your sleep needs will have changed over the course of your lifetime. You have to be prepared to adjust your expectations, and so your behavior, accordingly.

A particular problem with insomnia is that sleep is likely to be upset in a way that makes each night different. For example, a person with insomnia may sleep 3 or 4 hours some nights, while on other nights manage to get 6 or 7 hours. In one way or another, insomnia is often a mix of bad nights and better nights, which is pretty frustrating. Another common problem is that difficulties getting to sleep and waking in the night break the sleep that you do get into bits. This will make it feel as if you have had even less sleep, even if the total time, added up, doesn't look so bad.

I imagine that it may be hard for you to know how much sleep you need, especially if your pattern is all over the place. Here's what I suggest in my clinic as the best way to find out how much sleep you need:

Using your Sleep Diary it is quite easy to work out how much sleep you are getting, on average, at the moment. First, write down in the spaces in Box 8.1 the amount of time you think you actually slept in total for each of the last 10 nights. Second, add up the total time you have slept across these nights. Third, divide the total by 10 to get the *average length of your night's sleep.*

BOX 8.1 CALCULATING YOUR AVERAGE SLEEP TIME

Night
1
Amount of time I slept

_____

_____

Night
2
Amount of time I slept

_____

_____

Night
3

Amount of time I slept

_____

_____

Night
4
Amount of time I slept

_____

_____

Night
5
Amount of time I slept

_____

_____

Night
6
Amount of time I slept

_____

_____

Night
7
Amount of time I slept

_____

_____

Night
8
Amount of time I slept

_____

_____

_____

Night
9
Amount of time I slept

_____

_____

Night
10
Amount of time I slept

_____

_____

Total amount of sleep over 10 days=_____
My average sleep time=_____ /10=_____

Before we move on to the next step, it is worth saying that you will probably have come up with a figure that is less than what you are aiming at. But this is just your starting point. So far we have only found out how much sleep you are getting. Remember that no matter how little sleep that adds up to, it will still be worthwhile sleep.

Follow the program with me and you will see how you can first of all get rid of your difficulties getting to sleep and staying asleep, and after that you can build up your total sleep time to the amount of sleep you actually need.

Setting your time in bed

Your next goal is to work out a way of achieving the *same* amount of sleep *every* night. This is important because we should be aiming for a sleep pattern that you can rely upon – that is, one that is stable and does not vary much from night to night. We know that good sleepers can rely on having a consistent pattern, so this should be your goal, too.

We have found out the average amount of sleep that you have been getting. Now I want you to get this same amount every night, but in one continuous sleep. In other words, to get you sleeping right through!

Deciding on your rising time

I always recommend that you should *anchor* your sleep around a *fixed morning rising time.* This anchoring is to stop your sleep from drifting and to help it to settle down to a reliable pattern. To do this, you should now choose a time in the morning that you will rise from bed. The time you choose is up to you, but it should be a time that you are comfortable with and that allows you to do all the things you need to do during the day. For example, you may find that 6:30 or 7:00a.m. is a good time to set because during the week you need to get up then for work. Once you have decided, write this time down in Box 8.2.

You should now have both your average sleep time and your fixed morning rising time. The next thing to think about is when bedtime should be. At the moment, how do you decide when to go to bed?

BOX 8.2 RISING TIME

My morning rising time is _____

Deciding on your threshold time

Sometimes people go to bed before they are sleepy-tired and end up lying awake, or they fall asleep quickly but wake up very early. At other times, people will go to bed early to try to catch up on the sleep they have lost on previous nights. People sometimes say that they go to bed because 'everyone else has gone to bed', or just because 'it's bedtime.' People even force themselves to stay up very late in an effort to exhaust themselves, in the belief that this will make them sleep better.

However, the answer to the question 'When should I go to bed?' is fairly straightforward. You should go to bed at a time which makes it likely that you will sleep right through the night. The next step, then, is to set what I call a *threshold time* for going to bed. This is to mark the point at which you can cross the threshold from waking to sleeping. It is worked out by subtracting your average sleep time from your morning rising time.

Let me give you an example. Suppose someone has worked out that their average sleep time is 6 1/2 hours, and that they have set their rising time at 7:00a.m. By subtracting 6 1/2 hours from 7:00a.m. we get 12:30a.m. The threshold time for this person, then, is 12:30a.m. This person can then go to bed at this time, providing they feel sleepy-tired then. You should now work out your threshold time by following the steps in Box 8.3.

BOX 8.3 CALCULATING YOUR THRESHOLD TIME FOR CONSIDERING GOING TO BED

My threshold time is: _____

My average sleep time _____ – My set rising time _____ = _____

Please remember that your threshold time is *not* your actual bedtime. Your time for going to bed must always be at, or after, the threshold. Your threshold time is the *earliest* you can go to bed. I want you to monitor how sleepy-tired you feel and then to go to bed when you feel sleepy-tired and after you get to the threshold.

Summary of the sleep restriction program

I think there is a very good chance that you will now be seriously worried! What times have you arrived at? It is likely that either you will feel that it is very early to get up in the morning, or that it seems very late to stay up until your threshold time. Maybe you even think that both will be a major problem. It is important, therefore, that you do not forget that I am trying to help you get a new and consistent sleep pattern going.

I want to make sure, however, that you don't overdo things. Remember I said that sleep scheduling is based upon stimulus control and sleep restriction? Well, the bed/sleep connection advice I have given you is about the stimulus control part. Working out your sleep needs and your *sleep window* (when you can be in bed) is about sleep restriction. The goal is to maximize the chances that you will sleep right through. Sleep restriction is *not* the same as sleep deprivation. So, if you find from your Sleep Diary that your average sleep is less than 5 hours, I want you to work out your threshold time based on a *minimum of 5 hours in bed.*

You should now have all the information you need to decide on your new sleep schedule. Set the window to the size of your average sleep at the present time (or at 5 hours if your current average is less than 5 hours), and fix your morning rising time and threshold time. If you would rather not get up so early, then fix your rising time for a bit later – but also stay up later. If you would rather get to bed earlier, that is fine, too – but you have to rise earlier.

A nightly schedule

You may be thinking, 'Surely he doesn't mean that I have to do this *every* night, including weekends?' Sorry, the answer is yes. You're facing quite a challenge getting your sleep pattern sorted out, and it is going to take a *seven-nights-a-week* CBT treatment to do it. Your threshold time and your rising time are meant for *every* day of the week.

Let me explain a little more. The aim is to reset your sleep pattern and to increase your *sleep efficiency.* Remember that sleep efficiency is simply the percentage of time you spend in bed sleeping.

For example, Craig goes to bed at 11:00p.m., but does not fall asleep until 12:30a.m. He also is awake for 30 minutes in the middle of the night. So when Craig wakes up at 7:00a.m., he has slept for 6 hours but he has been in bed for 8 hours, having been awake for a total of 2 hours. Craig's sleep efficiency score is the number of hours he has slept (6) divided by the number of hours he has spent in bed (8), multiplied by 100. This gives him a sleep efficiency of only 75 per cent.

If you slept right through from the moment your head hit the pillow until the moment your alarm clock went off you would be sleeping 100 per cent of the night! The sleep-restriction program I have described for you actually gives you the chance of reaching that 100 per cent, at least some nights, because homeostatic pressure for sleep (your sleep drive) will build up as you follow the program every night. Sleep inevitably will fill in the only gap you make available to it – your new 'sleep window'. In practice, though, I want to help you to increase your sleep efficiency to around 90 per cent. That is an achievable goal. I accept that weekends will be hard for you, so use your alarm clock to make sure you rise at your fixed time.

I have summarized the sleep-scheduling component of the CBT program in Box 8.4 so that you can put it all together. You will see that I have added some questions to help you think about each instruction in practical terms. I suggest that you sit down with your notebook and write down your answers to each of these questions, and that you problem-solve any that are likely to pose a particular problem. If you have a partner or there are others in the house with you, it can be a good idea to discuss these solutions with them. I have found that people with insomnia are often worried, for example, about getting out of bed when they can't sleep, in case it disturbs the household. By discussing solutions with others involved I think you will find that they will often be happy to support you in trying to solve your sleep problem – whatever it takes.

BOX 8.4 SUMMARY OF THE SLEEP SCHEDULING PROGRAM

1 Stay up until your threshold time.

(When is that? How are you going to use your extra time in the evening?)

2 Lie down in bed only when you feel sleepy.

(What are your signs of sleepiness?)

3 Do not use your bed for anything except sleep.

(What changes are you going to have to make?)

4 If you do not get to sleep quickly (within 15 minutes), get up.

(What exactly will you do when you get up? What preparations do you need to make before you even go to bed?)

5 If you still cannot fall asleep, repeat Step 4.

(What exactly will you do?)

6 If you wake during the night, repeat Step 4.

216

> *(What exactly will you do?)*
> 7 Get up in the morning at your rising time.
> *(How will you make sure?)*
> 8 Do not nap during the day or evening right up to your threshold time.
> *(How are you going to make sure you avoid napping?)*
> 9 Follow this program seven days/nights a week.
> *(How will you manage this?)*

It feels like surgery!

I mentioned to you in Part One that I say to some patients with insomnia that I think their sleep problem is worse than they do! Requiring, if you like, special treatment. Well, here it is.

I know that the sleep scheduling is going to be tough for you. I sometimes call it 'the surgical option' because it is a bit like cutting out an old and malfunctioning part and implanting a replacement.

Changes can be difficult to put into practice, and they can be even harder to keep going. You may find that the first few nights are not too bad and that you manage without difficulty. However, you will definitely be tempted at times to forego the quarter-of-an-hour rule, for example.

It is at times like these that you have to make that extra effort and stick to your new sleep schedule. You have to remember that your insomnia is a tough problem to overcome, and that if the CBT program is to work for you, you have to follow it the way it was designed. I have to say that it is only by maintaining the changes you have put in place that your sleep pattern can be improved. So it is important that negative thoughts such as 'I am never going to get a good night's sleep' are replaced with more positive ones such as 'This problem is hard to break, but I am going to keep on following this program because it has been shown to be effective for people like me.' *Keeping motivated* is the key to achieving permanent changes in your sleep pattern.

The diagram I produced for you in Chapter 5 (Figure 5.2, p.89) showed you the process of making changes when it is hard to do so. Have another look at that now, and re-read that earlier section. Your motivation will come and go; that is to be expected. Relapses will occur some nights when you just can't follow the plan. These are times when you will experience a strong feeling of disappointment in yourself and think that there is no point trying again. Please don't let relapses discourage you. They are normal. The best thing to do is to get right back on course. I honestly think you may never have a better chance to sort out your sleep problems.

Making adjustments in sleep scheduling

'But am I going to get stuck with this short sleep window?' I hear you ask. I don't expect that you will get stuck. I hope that you will end up getting more sleep because, once your pattern adjusts, you can begin to lengthen the amount of time you spend in bed.

At first, the idea is that by restricting the amount of time you spend in bed you will be able to sleep right through. Instead of having bits of sleep, I want to see it all squashed together. But then we can let it grow a bit bigger, hopefully to the amount you would like ... or at least to the amount you need.

Your guide here, again, is your sleep efficiency. Once you are sleeping 90 per cent of the time you are in bed (threshold time to rising time) for one full week, you can increase your time in bed by 15 minutes for the next week, by either going to bed 15 minutes earlier or staying in bed 15 minutes later in the morning. After trying that out for the next week, you can check if you still make it to 90 per cent. If you do, then you can increase your sleep window by another 15 minutes. But please note you must be very strict and not go above

15 minutes per week at any time. You can make these adjustments several times perhaps, but you will come to the point when you are in fact sleeping as much as you need. At that point, trying to spend longer in bed will not give you any more sleep and you have achieved your established pattern. Here is an example:

Carolyn has been following a 6-hour sleep window and is now managing to sleep an average of 5 1/2 hours per night. When she does the arithmetic, her sleep efficiency is now over 90 per cent (5 5/6)x100=91.7 per cent. So, during the next week she can increase her sleep window to 6 hours and 15 minutes. She can either set her alarm for 15 minutes later, or she can go to bed 15 minutes earlier. She cannot do both. This new schedule can then be followed for a further week to see if she is able to sleep even longer.

Monitoring your sleep

I know that I keep reminding you about the importance of your Sleep Diary as you go through the program. Now you will see one of the reasons why. Your diary information is very valuable in making the adjustments you need to make. Remember to work on all the material you have covered in this chapter for a full week before going on to the next section.

9

Dealing with a racing mind (Program Week 5)

Introduction

So often people have said to me that their main problem is not being able to empty their mind ... not being able to stop their thoughts from racing. Sometimes they say that they feel physically exhausted but they just cannot seem to switch off mentally. Indeed, research studies have shown that people with insomnia are actually more aware of *mental* symptoms of arousal than they are of *bodily* (physiological) symptoms. I wouldn't be surprised, therefore, if you had flicked open to the Contents page of this book, spotted this chapter, and headed straight here.

Of course, as I keep reminding you, this is a course of treatment, a program of CBT. So I don't want you to pick and choose. Nevertheless, I am sure that many of you who are using the program will find this chapter particularly important and helpful too.

I am going to take you through the strategies that we teach our patients to deal with thoughts and worries related to sleep. I will also introduce some of the assessment measures that we use, so that you can sort out the type of thought problems you are having, and so can find suitable solutions.

Aim

The purpose of this session is *to learn ways of overcoming the mental alertness, repetitive thoughts and anxieties that interfere with your sleep.*

Knowing the enemy

As I was just saying, research has shown that people with insomnia complain a lot about an overactive mind in bed. They may or may not be the kind of people who have an overactive mind in the daytime, too. Some people seem to get into the habit of using their time in bed as a time to think things through. Maybe they lead busy daytime lives and just run out of thinking time! Others find that it is impossible to keep their minds empty when it is quiet and they can't sleep, and then they get preoccupied with their own thoughts – however important or trivial they may be. The busy and racing mind is the enemy of sleep.

First of all, then, let's consider the kinds of things that you think about when you are in bed and unable to get to sleep. There are several types of thoughts that are common, so I want you to consider each of these to see if they ring a bell.

Rehearsing and planning thoughts

As the name suggests, this is when you think back over the day or recent events, or when you look ahead to things that are about to come up. Replaying the day's events at the end of the day is in some ways quite a natural thing to do. Perhaps it is even enjoyable at times! It just so happens that the night separates one day from the next, so at the close of the day it is normal to reflect on what you did and on how things went. Likewise, thinking ahead to the next day and planning ahead to future events may be on your mind. Tomorrow is, after all, a new day, with all its activities and responsibilities. You may find you go into checklist mode. If so, you are likely to find yourself anticipating, either positively or negatively, the day ahead. My point is that your rehearsing and planning thoughts might keep you awake simply because they cause mental alertness in bed.

Problem-solving thoughts

You may have things on your mind because you think this or that 'needs to get sorted out'. This kind of thought pushes itself to the front of your mind because it carries with it a sense of urgency. There's a problem, or at least a perceived problem, and you must find a solution. So you stay awake while you try to come up with an answer. It could be that you are able to keep things in the back of your mind during the day, but at night, because you are not occupied with other things, these thoughts begin to dominate. These thoughts often require some concentrated attention because there may be options to think through properly before you can make a decision or a plan. That's why they are really best dealt with during the day, when you are awake. If *problem-solving* is part of your night-time routine, little wonder that you have difficulty sleeping. In this type of thinking there's no doubt that your mind will actually be working quite hard. So it's a recipe for staying awake, because when we are tired and cranky we really don't solve problems very well. Then, of course, we realize that we are not coming up with a good solution, which makes us get caught up all the more in mental and emotional alertness.

Thinking about sleeping

You may feel that you don't really have any problems ... except the insomnia problem! *Thinking about sleeping,* or more likely, thinking about the fact that you're *not* sleeping, is very much part of every insomnia problem. It's part of the vicious circle – I want to sleep – I can't sleep – I can't stop thinking about wanting to sleep – so I'm keeping myself awake. When sleep doesn't come quickly or naturally you may well find that you become preoccupied with your sleeplessness. But there is probably more to it than that. You begin to think about the *consequences* of not sleeping. 'How am I going to get through tomorrow?', 'If I don't get to sleep soon I will only have had a few hours sleep,' and so on. These kinds of thoughts often lead us to try too hard to get to sleep.

Listening to your body

This is a bit like the last one. What I mean by *listening to your body* is that you start to focus inwards and notice how tired you are, or how awake you are. Maybe you can't stop listening to your heart beat; it thumps away in your ear as you lie on your side in bed. Or some other body sensation like feeling hot or cold, or an annoying itch, or restlessness in your legs, or muscle tension. You get the idea

– you are 'tuned into' your body, as if you are undertaking a detailed observational study of yourself. This kind of thinking can make us very restless in bed. Thinking about your health would come into this category too, especially after a period of illness, when it is quite natural to find that you are preoccupied with your health. These are all examples of *self-awareness* thoughts, when your mind is quite concentrated and focused, and is not good for getting off to sleep.

Thinking about thinking

This is quite an important one because, many times, people with insomnia are at pains to point out that they *don't* have worries or depression and that everything really is fine. The frustrating thing for them is that they know that the thoughts keeping them awake are absolutely trivial. Do you do this *thinking about thinking* sometimes? When your mind buzzes around, darting from idea to idea? Usually the ideas, thoughts or images are silly or unimportant, and you might then think 'Why on earth did that come into my head?' The trivial nature of these thoughts can then become a focus in itself because it is intensely frustrating to feel that you are dominated by nonsensical or unimportant thoughts. Commonly, with these types of thoughts you may feel that you can't control your thinking, even though you are not really worrying about anything. Feeling that control is slipping away is not good for relaxing into sleep.

Thinking about things that go bump in the night

I would say that this is really not a major feature of insomnia, but it does sometimes happen that people become anxious or preoccupied by things in their environment at night. I don't really mean ghouls and ghosts, just that sometimes people can't get to sleep because of noises they hear, or think they hear. The wind outside, people in the street, an unfamiliar sound that you can't explain to yourself – because your senses home in on what you have noticed (you may even hold your breath to listen more intently), it becomes very hard to sleep.

Thoughts and emotions

It is not very realistic to try to separate our thoughts from our emotions. I would advise you to consider how you are feeling as well as what you are thinking. Our mind is a *combination* of thoughts and feelings. Maybe there are worries in your life at the moment, about family, work, health, money or whatever.

So when you are having your rehearsing, planning type of thoughts, or your problem-solving thoughts, you may find that you get strong emotional feelings. Of course, the thoughts plus the feelings keep you even more awake. Disappointment, sadness, guilt, frustration, and worry in our thoughts make sleep so much more difficult. If you are feeling emotionally drained or strained, it may be even harder to deal with your lack of sleep. It is, of course, important to work out if there is a separate problem with your emotions that needs help in its own right. The CBT program can help your insomnia, and that will surely help how you feel, but remember that it is not a treatment for depression or for other emotional or mental health problems.

On the other hand, I am not trying to imply that you do have a serious emotional problem. I believe people when they say they have nothing to worry about; even lots to be grateful for. You may not be unhappy or anxious in your life or with yourself in a general sense. So it is particularly frustrating when you can't find the final piece of the jigsaw. Certainly, not being able to get to sleep does get us emotional. At times your frustration may even turn to annoyance or anger. You lie there thinking about how you can't get to sleep, perhaps knowing that you are keeping yourself awake. You are actually winding yourself up emotionally!

Measuring the content of your thoughts

I hope this is helping you to 'assess the enemy'. To help you a bit more I have reproduced for you in Figure 9.1 as a simple rating scale called the Glasgow Content of Thoughts Inventory (GCTI). This came from work we have done with people with insomnia, which helped us to find out the most common thoughts that were in their minds as they tried to fall asleep. The best way to use the scale may be to photocopy it so you can use it more than once.

You just follow the instructions and give a rating for each item. That will give you a profile of the kinds of thoughts that interfere most often with your sleep. You will see that you can also add up the scores to a total score and to three sub-scores. The three sub-scores are items that relate to one another under a general heading. You can calculate, using these, which area or areas you have the most problem with. Spend a little time completing the GCTI now.

Another use of the GCTI would be to fill it in every few weeks to see if your scores are getting any lower. Think of the GCTI as giving you target areas to work on, and also as a way of measuring your progress in tackling these targets.

OK, so we have spent quite a bit of time on trying to understand and measure the types of thoughts that may be causing you some trouble. What can we do to overcome a racing mind?

Can I make the first strike?

I'm sticking with the analogy of a battle, because I think that's the way people often experience it! What do I mean by a *first strike?* I mean a pre-emptive one. By getting in first, before thoughts and anxieties have the potential to disrupt your night, you might be able to save yourself quite a bit of upset.

Putting the day to rest

I think you may find this technique particularly useful for thoughts that have to do with the past day and thoughts relating to planning for the following day. The aim is to put the day to bed, along with all your plans for the next day, long before bedtime ... so that when bedtime comes you can get to sleep. If you can manage to deal with the kind of thinking that you usually do in bed before it happens, then you should sleep better.

Figure 9.1 The Glasgow Content of Thoughts Inventory (GCTI)

Here are some thoughts that people have when they cannot sleep.

Please indicate, by placing a tick in the appropriate box, how often over the past 7 nights the following thoughts have kept you awake.

Thought
1 Events in the future
Never 0

_____

_____

Sometimes 1

_____

_____

Often 2

_____

_____

Always 3

_____

_____

Thought
2 Hew tired/sleepy you feel
Never 0

_____

_____

Sometimes 1

Often 2

Always 3

Thought
3 What happened during the day
Never 0

Sometimes 1

Often 2

Always 3

Thought
4 How nervous/anxious you feel

Never 0

Sometimes 1

Often 2

Always 3

Thought
5 How mentally awake you feel
Never 0

Sometimes 1

Often 2

Always 3

Thought
6 Checking the lime
Never 0

Sometimes 1

Often 2

Always 3

Thought
7 Trivial things
Never 0

Sometimes 1

Often 2

_____

_____

Always 3

_____

_____

Thought
8 How you can't stop your mind from racing
Never 0

_____

_____

Sometimes 1

_____

_____

Often 2

_____

_____

Always 3

_____

_____

Thought
9 How long you've been awake
Never 0

Sometimes 1

Often 2

Always 3

Thought
10 Your health
Never 0

Sometimes 1

Often 2

Always 3

236

Thought
11 Ways you can get to sleep
Never 0

Sometimes 1

Often 2

Always 3

Thought
12 Things you have to do tomorrow
Never 0

Sometimes 1

Often 2

_____

_____

Always 3

_____

_____

Thought
13 How hot/cold you feel
Never 0

_____

_____

Sometimes 1

_____

_____

Often 2

_____

_____

Always 3

_____

_____

Thought
14 Your work/responsibilities
Never 0

_____

_____

_____

Sometimes 1

_____

_____

_____

Often 2

_____

_____

_____

Always 3

_____

_____

_____

Thought
15 How frustrated/annoyed you feel
Never 0

_____

_____

_____

Sometimes 1

_____

_____

_____

Often 2

_____

_____

_____

Always 3

Thought
16 How light/dark the room is
Never 0

Sometimes 1

Often 2

Always 3

Thought
17 Noises you hear
Never 0

Sometimes 1

Often 2

_____

_____

Always 3

_____

_____

Thought
18 Being awake all night
Never 0

_____

_____

Sometimes 1

_____

_____

Often 2

_____

_____

Always 3

_____

_____

Thought
19 Pictures of things in your mind
Never 0

Sometimes 1

Often 2

Always 3

Thought
20 The effects of not sleeping well
Never 0

Sometimes 1

Often 2

Always 3

Thought
21 Your personal life
Never 0

Sometimes 1

Often 2

Always 3

Thought
22 How thinking too much is the problem
Never 0

Sometimes 1

Often 2

_____

_____

_____

Always 3

_____

_____

_____

Thought
23 Things in your past
Never 0

_____

_____

_____

Sometimes 1

_____

_____

_____

Often 2

_____

_____

_____

Always 3

_____

_____

_____

Thought
24 How had you are at sleeping
Never 0

Sometimes 1

Often 2

Always 3

Thought
25 Things to do to help you sleep
Never 0

Sometimes 1

Often 2

Always 3

Total score: add items 1 to 25 (note the maximum score is 75)

Subscale 1: focusing on rehearsing/planning/problem-solving.

Add items 1, 3, 8, 12, 14, 15, 19, 21 and 23.

Subscale 2: focusing on your sleep and wakefulness.

Add items 5, 6, 7, 9, 11, 18, 22, 24 and 25.

Subscale 3: focusing on your self and sensory awareness.

Add items 2, 4, 10, 13, 16, 17 and 20.

I call this technique *putting the day to rest.* Here is what is involved. Simply follow the steps I have summarized in Box 9.1. Twelve steps may seem a lot, but honestly you can do this in 20 minutes, no problem. You just have to make the time and get into the discipline of putting the day to rest before the evening really gets going. Remember that the thoughts that interfere at bedtime will be so much easier to dismiss if they have already been dealt with ... at a time when you were much more awake.

Using your knowledge to combat worry

I hope you have been getting better at using what you now know to evaluate your thoughts and attributions. This is just a reminder to keep using those techniques I taught you before. Are you remembering to use your thought-evaluation form (Table 6.2, p.111)? Your outlook upon your sleep and your attitude towards sleeplessness are so important. These things are also part of your pre-emptive strike force. *You* are in charge of the amount of damage that a poor night's sleep can do to you, because a lot of that depends on your *perspective.* I would encourage you to re-read that section of the book at this point.

BOX 9.1 PUTTING THE DAY TO REST

1 Set aside 20 minutes in the early evening, the same time every night if possible (say around 7p.m.).

2 Sit down somewhere you are not going to be disturbed.

3 All you need is a notebook, your diary, and a pen.

4 Think of what has happened during the day, how events have gone, and how you feel about the kind of day it has been.

5 Write down some of the main points. Put them to rest by committing them to paper. Write down what you feel good about and also what has troubled you.

6 Write down anything you feel you need to do on a 'to do' list with steps that you can take to tie up any loose ends or unfinished business.

7 Now think about tomorrow and what's coming up. Consider things you are looking forward to as well as things that may cause you worry.

8 Write down your schedule in your diary, or check it if it's already there.

9 Write down anything you are unsure about and make a note in your diary of a time in the morning when you are going to find out about that.

10 Try to use your 20 minutes to leave you feeling more in control. Close the book on the day.

11 When it comes to bedtime, remind yourself that you have already dealt with all these things if they come into your mind.

12 If new thoughts come up in bed, note them down on a piece of paper at your bedside to be dealt with the following morning.

Turning the tide

Of course you need tools to help you when you are in bed, too. Here are some of the ones that are most effective for my patients.

Thought-blocking

I have found that people with insomnia find this technique works best with the trivial, less important thoughts rather than with more worrying or more serious problems. Sometimes trivial interrupting thoughts come to people when they wake up in the middle of the night. When this happens, it is best to start the thought-blocking immediately upon waking before you get too wide awake! Thought-blocking involves following the three simple steps I have summarized in Box 9.2.

BOX 9.2 THREE STEPS TO SUCCESSFUL THOUGHT-BLOCKING

1 Repeat the word 'the' every 2 seconds in your head with your eyes closed.

2 Don't say it out loud, but it sometimes helps to 'mouth' it.

3 Keep up the repetitions for about 5 minutes (if you can!).

Thought-blocking works by stopping other thoughts from getting in. As the term suggests, it creates a block. But why should this work? Well, the word 'the' is, of course, meaningless. So when you repeat it to yourself it doesn't have *any* emotional effect, except maybe to bore you ... and that might actually help!

Let me give you an illustration of how a small amount of information repeated to yourself can stop other information getting in. Suppose you have looked in the telephone directory to find a number to call, but the phone book is in one room and the telephone is in another. You decide just to try to remember the number, so you walk to the phone rehearsing the number over and over to yourself. As you walk through the hallway, someone in your family is there and just says 'Hi'. What happens? You really can't respond, you can hardly even look at them ... because your total mental capacity is taken up with repeating just a few numbers.

Give the thought-blocking technique a good try and see how you get on with it. Thinking the word 'the' to yourself slowly and calmly every two seconds really helps you disconnect not only from the outside world, but importantly, also from your own thought processes.

Relaxation and Imagery

During Week 2 of this program you learned about how to use a relaxation routine. Relaxation is a good way of relaxing the mind, as well as the body. This is because it is a pretty good *distraction technique.* It helps you focus your mind away from intrusive and worrying thoughts. I think it may help you deal with the kind of thoughts that dart around all over the place. Relaxation exercises can give you more of a sense of being in control – of your breathing, your muscles, your mind. It is in this sense a good tool to have in life as a coping response whenever you feel under pressure.

What I want to do now is introduce something called *imagery.* This can be bolted on quite easily to your relaxation exercises. Imagery involves creating a mental picture, a kind of visual story in your mind. I would imagine many of you will have tried this when you can't get to sleep at night. You try thinking of something pleasant, maybe a peaceful place you know, or a holiday you enjoyed somewhere. The old idea of counting sheep and watching them jump the gate is an example of imagery. So this is the general principle of what I mean, but there is evidence to suggest that this kind of 'thinking something up' imagery is not very effective. Maybe you have found that too?

The research data tell us that, in order to be effective, imagery should be *planned* in advance and should be well *practised.* Some of the essentials for imagery training can be found in Box 9.3.

BOX 9.3 THE ESSENTIALS OF IMAGERY TRAINING

- **Be prepared** – don't just wait until the time comes and try to think something up. Develop a screenplay! You are the director, so shoot the scenes and edit them until you have got what you want. Your imagery sequence should take about 10 minutes to go through in your mind's eye.
- **Practice regularly** – you are also a participant! You must learn the scenes and the sequences so that they flow as the movie rolls! You need to set time aside to learn the 'script' and you should practice in the evening or during the day too.
- **Get good quality images** – vivid and clear in your mind's eye is what you want. Notice the colours, the smells, the sounds, the sensations that you make part of your imagery routine.
- **Relax and enjoy!** – who wants to watch a movie that is uninteresting? This is something that you should look forward to. But at the same time remember you want to develop an imagery story that is calming,

soothing, and not evocative of strong emotions!

I suggest that you follow your relaxation routine and then follow straight through into your own imagery story. You can also practice joining them up. As you get better at using imagery you will find that it is another good distractor from unwanted intrusive thoughts and emotions because it captures your attention.

Sleep scheduling

You have already begun to establish a new sleep habit because you are following the sleep-scheduling part of the program. Why am I mentioning sleep scheduling in this section too? Simply because many of these behavioral rules are also very effective against a racing mind.

For example, staying up until you are sleepy-tired means that you are more likely to fall asleep quickly rather than lying awake thinking. In the same way, getting out of bed if you are awake for quarter of an hour means that you will have less thinking time in bed ... and that is a very good thing! Remember we spoke about building up a strong bed/sleep connection. The sleep-scheduling program will help you remove thoughts and emotions that occur at night into another part of the house.

This should mean that sleep is less interrupted by your mental overactivity. So keep up the good sleep-scheduling work that you have already started!

Giving up trying to sleep

Sometimes people are unable to sleep because they are simply trying too hard. We spoke before about *sleep attention, sleep intention* and *sleep effort* in this regard. Trying to fall asleep actually keeps you wakeful and leads to irritability when you don't succeed. It is understandable that you want to sleep and then try to make it happen. The drawback is that, unlike many other things in life, sleep is not something that you can *make* happen by sheer force of will. In fact, the harder you try, the less likely it is to happen. But how do you give up trying to sleep? I have found that two methods work; you can decide which of them suits you best (Table 9.1). You may think, looking at Table 9.1 above, that I have finally taken leave of my senses! But if there is a madness in my method, there is also a method in my madness! Let me explain.

TABLE 9.1: METHODS FOR GIVING UP TRYING TO SLEEP
Method 1: Turn the tables

- Take every opportunity to be carefree about your insomnia.

Method 2: Try to stay awake

- Lie comfortably in your bed with the lights off, but keep your eyes open.

Method 1: Turn the tables

- Relish opportunities to get out of bed whenever you can.

Method 2: Try to stay awake

- Give up any effort to fall asleep.

Method 1: Turn the tables

- Try to imagine as many catastrophes as you can that will happen, just because you are awake at night. See them as exaggerated and absurd.

Method 2: Try to stay awake

- Give up any concern about still being awake.

Method 1: Turn the tables

- Be prepared to accept you have insomnia. Even tell others about it.

Method 2: Try to stay awake

- When your eyelids feel like they want to close, say to yourself gently 'Just stay awake for another couple of minutes, I'll fall asleep naturally when I'm ready.'

Method 1: Turn the tables

- Think of wakefulness as an opportunity, not a disaster. Use the time when you are up, to do something useful or something you enjoy.

Method 2: Try to stay awake
• Don't purposefully make yourself stay awake; but if you can shift the focus off attempting to fall asleep, you will find that sleep comes naturally.

The use of *humour* is extremely powerful in helping us to take a different perspective. If we need to *de-catastrophize* a situation, that is, to reduce all our exaggerated conclusions and emotions, then humour presents a good way forward. This is in part what I mean by 'turning the tables'. Try to think 'What is the worst that can happen?' and then challenge the true likelihood of all your wild imaginings. Try going with the flow instead of against it by posing less resistance to wakefulness. Accept that you will just get up if you are awake. Big deal – so do something with your extra time!

This is Method 1. It may or may not appeal to you, but I hope that you can see that a more light-hearted approach could help to reduce anxiety and effort around sleep. Patients using this approach often talk about developing a completely different attitude. Indeed, the idea of accepting situations rather than fighting them all the time has its roots in a number of ancient philosophies and religions. *Acceptance* leads to a problem having a less dominating position. Where sleep is concerned, a more mellow perspective is an adaptive outlook, and one that can lead to improved sleep.

Method 2 is an even more *paradoxical* method. In psychology we use this term to describe therapies where you are encouraged (paradoxically) to keep the symptom going, rather than trying to eliminate it. With insomnia you change your goal to that of staying awake, instead of getting to sleep. By deciding to stay awake you are *completely giving up trying* to sleep. When that happens you find yourself falling asleep in spite of yourself. How reassuring it can be to find that you are overtaken by sleep: 'I don't know what happened last night, I was trying to stay awake just a few minutes longer and the next thing I knew it was morning.' That is the kind of thing that patients say when this method works for them.

Making less of an effort

The two methods in Table 9.1 have the same goal – to help you give up trying to sleep. Letting sleep strengthen and develop again naturally will take you closer to your goal of being a good sleeper. The Glasgow Sleep Effort Scale (GSES) is a way of summarizing and scoring the sleep effort problem. I have reproduced the GSES for you in Figure 9.2.

Figure 9.2 The Glasgow Sleep Effort Scale

The following seven statements relate to your night-time sleep pattern *in the past week.*

Please indicate by circling one response how true each statement is for you.

Score 0 for 'not at all', 1 for 'to some extent' and 2 for 'very much', then add up your total score (maximum is 14)

1 I put too much effort into sleeping at night when it should come naturally.

Very much

To some extent

Not at all

2 I feel I should be able to control my sleep at night.

Very much

To some extent

Not at all

3 I put off going to bed at night for fear of not being able to sleep.

Very much

To some extent

Not at all

4 I worry about not sleeping if I am in bed at night and cannot sleep.

Very much

To some extent

Not at all

5 I am no good at sleeping at night.
Very much
To some extent
Not at all
6 I get anxious about sleeping before I go to bed at night.
Very much
To some extent
Not at all
7 I worry about the long-term consequences of not sleeping at night.
Very much
To some extent
Not at all

Why don't you fill it out just now, to represent the way you *usually* feel about your sleep? Hopefully you will see that the items in the scale reflect the habit of *sleep preoccupation* and *sleep effort* I have been talking about. Do you see from your score how over-involved you have become with your sleep? Now ask someone you know who is a good sleeper to fill it out. See what they score and make the comparison. Good sleep is pretty much effort-free!

I would like you to reduce your effortful approach to an effort-free approach by using Methods 1 or 2 (or both), and of course by keeping going with all the other parts of the CBT program. You can always fill the GSES in again at some point to see if you are getting closer to becoming a good sleeper!

Are you paying attention?

Do you remember the story about my car having a blown headlight, and then my noticing all the oncoming vehicles that also had one of their headlights out? That was a story about *attentional bias.* My focus of attention had been directed, without me really being aware of it. We drew parallels with the sleep attentional bias in insomnia. So how can you reduce your unhelpful focus on sleep and sleeplessness?

First of all let me say that many of the techniques we have covered will help with this. Feeling more prepared by putting the day to rest and having a pre-bedtime routine means that the prospect of sleep is less threatening because you will feel more in control. Relaxation, imagery, and thought-stopping give you distraction methods away from the focus on insomnia. The sleep-scheduling techniques will lead you to spend less time lying awake in bed aware of not being asleep. Have another skim-read back over the techniques I have recommended, and figure out for yourself how *CBT draws attention away from concern about insomnia.*

Chief among additional things that might help is abandoning *clock-watching.* So many

260

people over the years have said to me things like 'I see every hour' or 'When I wake up and look at the clock, I can't believe it's only (whatever time).' People with insomnia use clocks, not just to tell the time, but as performance indicators! They are part of the *self-monitoring tendency* that heightens wakefulness in bed and usually leads to negative self-evaluation.

TABLE 9.2: THE PROBLEM OF CLOCK-WATCHING

Awareness of time
'Look at that, it's gone 12:30...'
Dysfunctional thought
'...and I should be well asleep by now'
Self-evaluation
I have failed
Emotional response
Annoyance
Awareness of time
'I've been lying awake for almost 2 hours now and only caught a few minutes' sleep...'
Dysfunctional thought
'...if I don't sleep soon I'll be wrecked tomorrow'
Self-evaluation
I have lost control
Emotional response
Anxiety
Awareness of time

> 'Awake again ... so what's the time now? ... great (!) 4 a.m....'
> **Dysfunctional thought**
> '...I can't stand this any more; I'm going to go mad'
> **Self-evaluation**
> I can't cope
> **Emotional response**
> Despair

Here is the kind of scenario I am thinking of in Table 9.2. Can you see how the clock becomes a trigger that ends up with an emotional response that is arousing? Your awareness of time often gets linked to an automatic and dysfunctional thought. Because these thoughts usually contain verbs that carry a value judgement (like 'I *should...*') the next consequence is that you will evaluate yourself negatively, and this leads to a strong emotional response.

There are three solutions to clock-watching. The first two suggestions are fairly obvious. The advantage of removing the clock is that you are not so tempted to take a peek. The advantage of turning it away is that you can, when appropriate, make occasional time checks. An example of this is using the quarter-of-an-hour rule. You are not meant to monitor time exactly, but on the other hand I don't want you to create an excuse for lying awake for ages before you get up! The final possibility is that by not allowing the clock to trigger negative thoughts you could decide to challenge your usual *automatic thought* and your *self-evaluation.* Try to take an alternative perspective that is less upsetting and arousing. We have spoken about appraising your thoughts more accurately, and this is another opportunity to change the way that you think. I would recommend the combination of turning the clock away and using the trigger differently for starters, and see how you get on.

Evaluating how you feel in the day

Have another look at your scores on the Glasgow Content of Thoughts Inventory. I want you to have a particularly close look at items that relate to the links you make between your sleep and how you feel in the daytime. Items 12, 14, and 20 are examples. How did you score on these? Do you think that a major part of your insomnia problem lies in how you feel in the daytime following a poor night's sleep?

There are two solutions to this that I can think of, so you should probably use both. *Optimizing your sleep pattern* means following the CBT program, particularly sleep scheduling, as best as you can. You can be confident that as your sleep improves, benefits to your daytime life will follow! If you want to measure what I mean by this idea of optimizing, I suggest you check again on your sleep efficiency. Remember that this tells you about the percentage of time you spend in bed asleep. So, keep working on improving your sleep efficiency.

The second part of the solution is *evaluating your beliefs.* You need to be willing to question the conclusions you draw about *why* you are not at your best in the daytime. I'm not saying that it's nothing to do with your insomnia – but there might be other factors too. You need to find out about those. Have a look back this time to the sleep quiz at the start of Part Two. The answers I gave to questions 6, 7, 10, and 12 might help you here. Also keep using Table 6.2 and remind yourself of the examples I gave you in Table 6.1.

Making adjustments

While we are on the subject of sleep efficiency, this is a good time to remind you about the rules for adjusting your sleep schedule week by week. Remember your sleep efficiency is the key here, too. If after this week you are sleeping 90 per cent of the time you are in bed (threshold time to rising time), then you can increase your time in bed by 15 minutes for next week. You can either go to bed 15 minutes earlier or you can stay in bed 15 minutes longer in the morning.

Monitoring your sleep

Another gentle reminder about the importance of continuing to use your Sleep Diary. I hope you are seeing progress as you follow the whole CBT program. Work away at the materials in this chapter for one week before moving on to Chapter 10.

10

Putting it all together (Program Week 6)

Introduction

Well, I have covered most of the CBT materials now. This week's program is very much about learning how to put it all together and keep it together. Of course, I have emphasized this on the way through, but in this final week (Week 6) I want to illustrate how an integrated program can be achieved.

I would also point out that, although this is the last week of the program, you need to persevere for as long as it takes to overcome your insomnia and to become a good sleeper!

Aim

The purpose of this week is *to put together all the advice from the previous weeks and to help you to keep going with the program.*

Don't pick and choose

Try not to turn your nose up at things before you have really found out if they work for you. Some parts of CBT may at first look a bit unattractive, even a bit unsavoury. But an acquired taste is no bad thing, especially if it is good for your health, and especially your sleep.

Apologies if I have overdone the food analogy, but if you only remember the message because it is 'corny' I don't mind too much. I do want you to follow my recommendations, so here they are – all 32 of them! And these ingredients are *all* intended for you.

The CBT program in brief

You may want to photocopy Box 10.1 as a reminder of what we have covered. This is your *step-by-step summary* for implementing CBT to overcome insomnia. I think it speaks for itself.

Developing a confident approach

A good sleep pattern may take quite a number of weeks to establish. You must be prepared for this. It is important, therefore, that you recognize the progress you are making along the way. There are two ways of measuring progress. First, are you getting better at *implementing* the program? If so you are definitely making progress! Second, is your *sleep pattern* improving? You won't get the second without the first, so let's start with the implementation part.

Use the first column in Table 10.1 to write down what you have achieved so far. The simplest way would be to note down the item numbers (1 to 32) that you are now managing to put into practice. Put the date at the top of the sheet, so you know where you stand right now. You can fill it in again in a couple of weeks and make a comparison, so again you might want to make a copy of Table 10.1 or put the information in your notebook instead.

I know from experience that it won't be all good news. So write down the item numbers that are still not achieved (or not fully achieved) in the second column. Everyone finds some parts of the program more difficult than others. Don't be too discouraged by that. Instead, let's consider the reasons why.

BOX 10.1 OVERVIEW OF THE CBT PROGRAM FOR OVER-COMING INSOMNIA

Some basics:
• Think of insomnia as a bad habit that can be corrected and stick to the program until you establish a good habit.

- Consider gradually reducing any sleeping pills that you take, but consult your physician first to agree a plan.
- Get a comfortable bed and mattress suitable to your needs and preferences.
- Work out your sleep schedule, your average sleep length, your planned rising time and threshold time for considering going to bed. Threshold time can be calculated by subtracting the average duration of your sleep at present from your planned rising time.
- Always follow your planned sleep schedule 7 nights a week.
- Make adjustments to your schedule at a maximum rate of 15 minutes per week and only after your sleep efficiency, the proportion of time spent asleep when in bed, reaches 90 per cent.

Before you go to bed:

1 Take light exercise in the late afternoon or early evening.

2 Put the day to rest long before bedtime. Think it through, tie up 'loose ends' in your mind and plan ahead. A notebook and diary will help to record and plan.

3 Wind down during the evening. Do not do anything mentally challenging within 90 minutes of bedtime, and stick to a routine.

4 Do not sleep or nap in the armchair. Keep sleep for bedtime.

5 Do not drink too much coffee or tea; eat a light snack for dinner and avoid eating chocolate and other products containing caffeine. Try to get used to de-caffeinated drinks.

6 Cut down your smoking in the evening and try not to smoke if you wake during the night.

7 Do not drink alcohol to aid your sleep – it usually upsets sleep.

8 Make sure your bed and bedroom are comfortable – not too cold, warm, noisy or bright. The room should be well aired and the alarm clock turned towards the wall.

9 Make preparations for waking during the night, such as leaving the heating on low in the living room and making a flask of a warm milky drink.

At bedtime:

10 Stay out of bed until your threshold time and until you feel 'sleepy-tired' – a tiredness that will make you fall asleep quickly and take you through the night.

11 Once in bed switch the light off immediately.

12 Do not read, watch TV, speak on the telephone, eat, drink, etc. in bed. The bedroom is for sleeping only, with the exception of sexual activity.

13 Practice relaxation exercises, followed by your imagery story. These procedures should be practised in the daytime before you try to apply them at night.

14 Give up trying to sleep. Keep your eyes open and gently resist sleep, or adopt a carefree or accepting attitude to wakefulness.

15 Remind yourself that sleep will come naturally. Repeat steps 13 and 14 as required.

16 Have your alarm set for the same rising time every day, 7 days a week, and make sure you rise at this time.

If you can't sleep or if you wake:

17 If you can't sleep within quarter of an hour of putting the light out, get up and go into the living room.

18 Use the same rule above if you wake during the night and can't get back to sleep quickly.

19 Do something relaxing (planned beforehand) for a while when out of bed and do not worry about tomorrow.

20 Remind yourself that sleep problems are common and not as damaging as you think. Try to avoid getting upset or frustrated.

21 Challenge all other intrusive and inaccurate ideas and mental images. Evaluate them and try to prevent them from dominating your thoughts.

22 Go back to bed when you feel 'sleepy-tired' again. Put the light out and relax.

23 Try to block out unwanted thoughts by repeating the word 'the' to yourself every 2 seconds. Try to keep this up for 5 minutes at a time.

24 Write down any intrusive thoughts or concerns in a notebook kept at your bedside and deal with them in the morning.

25 If you still can't sleep then get up again after quarter of an hour and repeat steps 19 to 24.

One possibility is that some of the advice may not be particularly relevant for you. If that is the case, then you can shift that item number into the third column. For example, maybe you never drink coffee, or don't have naps in the daytime anyway. Perhaps you don't have any problem falling asleep, so some of the things to do at bedtime don't seem necessary. If this is the kind of reason then it won't matter too much. But just be sure you are not cheating with the items you are putting into column three.

Another possibility is that you can't quite get a grip of some part of what you are meant to be doing. My advice here would be to go back and re-read the relevant sections of the book, and discuss anything you are confused about with someone you trust. I hope that this will clarify any points for you.

A third reason may be simply that what you are being asked to do is hard. It may be hard to remember some part of the program because of old habits that are difficult to break, or it may be hard to motivate yourself to do something, or to stick at it. For example, it is not easy to get up out of bed if you don't fall asleep within a quarter of an hour, or to rise at the same time seven days a week. It can be very hard to change our behavior. Likewise, we have to be quite strong in our minds to challenge negative and pessimistic thoughts so that they become more accurate and more encouraging ... and it is not easy to give up trying to sleep!

You may feel a bit disheartened by the middle column where you have written down the list of items that you are a bit stuck with right now. All I can say is that I would be astonished if you were already managing to put all of the instructions into practice all of the time! So, well done for all that you *are* doing. Try to be encouraged rather than discouraged. Be firm but fair with yourself for what you have achieved. Nevertheless, you have an agenda there to work on. Why don't you set some goals for implementing the tricky bits? Use your notebook to record your goals.

I hope your confidence is building now that you have a program for overcoming your insomnia. I hope your confidence is growing, too, because your sleep has shown some improvement. Now would be a good time to revisit the goals you wrote down at the start for what you were wanting to achieve. Are you getting closer to your goals? Remember they were to be *achievable* and *measurable.* Now is also a good time to measure your progress. Have you been sticking at using your Sleep Diary?

Identifying and monitoring your progress

I thought it might help if you had a table to summarize some of your Sleep Diary measures and how they have been changing over time. Have a look at Table 10.2.

The first column is for your sleep as it was at the start. You can transfer that information from your very first Sleep Diary. The second column is for how your sleep is now; that is from your most recent diary. There are other columns that you can use in the future. In our research studies we do follow-ups at 1, 3, and 6 months; sometimes even at 12 months, after completion of CBT programs. By completing Table 10.2 you should be able to see the *relationship* between what you are doing in implementing the CBT program and your progress with your sleep.

Conducting this careful analysis of your sleep pattern and sleep quality will also help you see exactly where there has been some positive change, and exactly where there is still room for improvement. I would encourage you to use your notebook to write down some *maintenance goals* and some *improvement goals.*

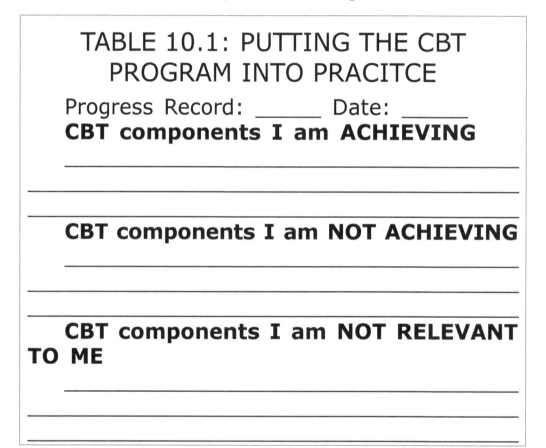

TABLE 10.1: PUTTING THE CBT PROGRAM INTO PRACITCE

Progress Record: _____ Date: _____

CBT components I am ACHIEVING

_____

_____

CBT components I am NOT ACHIEVING

_____

_____

CBT components I am NOT RELEVANT TO ME

_____

_____

Maintenance goals are your plans for keeping going with progress that has already taken place. For example, you might be falling asleep much more quickly now, so you want to make sure that you keep doing so. Your improvement goals would then be aspects of your sleep that still have some way to go. With the improvement goals, try to figure out how you can use the CBT program to help yourself. Write down in your notebook the conclusions you arrive at and the decisions you make about what to do. It may be that your record of putting CBT into practice (Table 10.1) will suggest things that need some extra work.

Trusting the evidence

You are now gathering your own *personal evidence* about CBT for insomnia, but I just want to remind you that there is a lot of *scientific evidence* indicating that CBT is likely to work for you. We know from studies that people keep on improving for at least six months after starting programs like this. In one of the studies that we did in Scotland we found continued improvement even a year later. Every encouragement, then, to keep on going! You will get more and more used to changes that you have made and you will reap more benefits. You have done the hard part so don't give up now.

Making lasting changes

Remember we are in this for the long game. I want to help you achieve change that will last. Ideally it would be great if you transformed from a poor sleeper to a good sleeper.

We have been concentrating on examining changes that may be seen in your sleep pattern itself, but I hope there will be more than this for you. People I see at my sleep clinics often report benefits to their general well-being, not just to their sleep. This is because sleeping well is healthy, and brings with it important bonuses. Improvements in concentration, productivity, mood and quality of life are certainly possible over a period of months. In my experience these form part of the changes that can last. Have a think about whether you are beginning to see any *generalized* benefits like these just now, and write these down in your diary.

TABLE 10.2: EVALUATING PROGRESS USING YOUR SLEEP DIARY

Sleep Diary measure
Wake-up time
Before CBT Date

_____

_____

Now Date

_____

_____

Follow-up Date

_____

_____

Follow-up Date

_____

_____

Follow-up Date

_____

Sleep Diary measure
Rising Time
Before CBT Date

_____

Now Date

_____

Follow-up Date

_____

Follow-up Date

_____

Follow-up Date

_____

_____

_____

Sleep Diary measure
Bedtime
Before CBT Date

_____

_____

Now Date

_____

_____

Follow-up Date

_____

_____

Follow-up Date

_____

_____

Follow-up Date

_____

_____

Sleep Diary measure
Lights out
Before CBT Date

_____

_____

Now Date

_____

_____

Follow-up Date

_____

_____

Follow-up Date

_____

_____

Follow-up Date

_____

_____

Sleep Diary measure
Time in bed (lights out to rising time: mins)

Before CBT Date

_____

_____

Now Date

_____

_____

Follow-up Date

_____

_____

Follow-up Date

_____

_____

Follow-up Date

_____

_____

Sleep Diary measure
Time to fall asleep (mins)
Before CBT Date

_____

_____

Now Date

_____

_____

Follow-up Date

_____

_____

Follow-up Date

_____

_____

Follow-up Date

_____

_____

Sleep Diary measure

Number of wakenings
Before CBT Date

_____

_____

Now Date

_____

_____

Follow-up Date

_____

_____

Follow-up Date

_____

_____

Follow-up Date

_____

_____

Sleep Diary measure
Time awake during wakenings (mins)
Before CBT Date

_____

_____

Now Date

_____

_____

Follow-up Date

_____

_____

Follow-up Date

_____

_____

Follow-up Date

_____

_____

Sleep Diary measure
Total time slept (mins)
Before CBT Date

_____

_____

Now Date

_____

_____

Follow-up Date

_____

_____

Follow-up Date

_____

_____

Follow-up Date

_____

_____

_____

Sleep Diary measure

Sleep efficiency (Total time slept/Time in bed x 100)

Before CBT Date

_____

_____

_____

Now Date

_____

_____

Follow-up Date

_____

_____

Follow-up Date

_____

_____

Follow-up Date

_____

_____

Sleep Diary measure

Sleeping pills (number or mg)

Before CBT Date

Now Date

Follow-up Date

Follow-up Date

Follow-up Date

Sleep Diary measure
Alcohol (units)
Before CBT Date

Now Date

Follow-up Date

_____

_____

Follow-up Date

_____

_____

Follow-up Date

_____

_____

Sleep Diary measure
Feeling rested after sleep 0, 1, 2, 3, or 4
Before CBT Date

_____

_____

Now Date

_____

_____

Follow-up Date

_____

_____

Follow-up Date

_____

_____

Follow-up Date

————————————

————————————

————————————

Sleep Diary measure
Sleep quality rating 0, 1, 2, 3, or 4
Before CBT Date

————————————

————————————

Now Date

————————————

————————————

Follow-up Date

————————————

————————————

Follow-up Date

————————————

————————————

Follow-up Date

————————————

————————————

————————————

You will encounter obstacles on the way, be sure of that. In my line of work we sometimes talk about something called *relapse-prevention*. Remember the wheel of motivation? It tells us that we should expect to slip at times, so it is best to be prepared for that. Sometime or other you will get some bad nights and you will worry that you are in danger of being back at 'square one'. Relapse-prevention tells you first to expect that to happen, and second to reinstate all the elements of the CBT program as soon as you can. If you feel that you are already doing these things and you can't understand why your sleep is disturbed, simply hold to your CBT course program, ride the storm, and it will probably rectify itself. Remember that acute sleep disturbance is essentially normal and temporary. It will tend to right itself as long as you don't get preoccupied with it.

You can also use this book as a form of *booster therapy.* This is a term we use in practice to describe how it often helps to give our progress a boost from time to time by refreshing the program. Just because you have read right through now doesn't mean that you have necessarily got the full benefit. Re-reading helps. Come back to the book to give yourself booster sessions on a regular basis. Why not even write some dates down right now in your notebook or your diary as a commitment to carrying on with the CBT approach?

Finally, keep in mind that your sleep efficiency is the key. I would urge you to check your sleep efficiency each and every week, aiming for 90 per cent. Make adjustments to your sleep window, as you have learned to do, and I am sure you will find that your sleep pattern becomes more regular and more satisfying. Once this happens you will be able to sleep without consciously using the CBT techniques or methods. They will have become second nature to you, and you will be well on the way to becoming a good sleeper.

My very best wishes to you in overcoming your insomnia.

PART THREE

Special Circumstances

Introduction to Part Three

The final part of this book comprises two brief chapters. They are relevant to you in the special circumstances where you may need to consider what to do either about sleep medication, or about the possibility that you have a sleep disorder other than insomnia. Chapter 11 is about sleeping pills and Chapter 12 is about what clinicians call 'differential diagnosis'.

11

What about sleeping pills?

Introduction

Although this book is about CBT, it is useful to include a brief chapter on sleeping pills. If you are taking medication for your insomnia, or are taking some other kind of medicine that affects your sleep, you must obtain advice from your prescribing doctor. I want to stress this point for two reasons. First, your doctor knows your overall physical and mental health and is best qualified to give advice about your medicine management. Second, the comments that I make here can only be taken as general in nature. They are *not* tailored to meet your particular individual needs. This chapter, therefore, should not be seen as an alternative to medical consultation.

Aim

The broad purpose of this chapter is *to assist you in considering what place sleeping pills have in your sleep-management plan.*

I don't believe in taking pills

Perhaps you have picked up this book because it is about CBT – which is a non-pharmacological approach to therapy. It may be that you are hoping to manage your sleep without using medication. Perhaps you prefer a non-drug approach to your health wherever that is possible.

Certainly, we live in an increasingly 'self-help' culture. If that means that people are becoming more and more interested in taking responsibility for their health, and for finding solutions to their health problems, then I think that is a very good thing. Indeed, I have written this book because I wanted to make available to people what I know to be an effective insomnia treatment.

However, I am not in any fundamental sense against a pharmacological approach. Rather, my standpoint is that there is ample sound scientific evidence for the effectiveness of CBT for *persistent insomnia.* By comparison, there is very little evidence to support the long-term use of sleeping pills for persistent insomnia. To me, this is a matter of *evidence-based clinical practice* and not a matter of principle or philosophy.

All the reviews of the evidence concerning sleeping pills come to the same conclusion: sleeping pills are not recommended for persistent sleep problems. However, they may be effective for acute or short-term insomnia. Taking a sleeping pill for a few nights, or for a couple of weeks, or from time to time, can be helpful to improve sleep over the short term. As far as I am aware, there are no guidelines anywhere in the world that recommend taking sleeping pills for months or for years.

I would rather not, but...

You may come to the matter of sleeping pills from the perspective that you would really rather not take sleeping pills, but that you have found that they have given you at least some relief from insomnia. Perhaps it is difficult not to take them, especially in the absence of any real alternative. Well hopefully, this CBT program will give you that alternative approach!

I have to acknowledge that it would be so much simpler if there was a sleeping pill that did the trick. CBT for insomnia involves quite a lot of hard work on your part ... and it has taken me all of these pages to explain it to you! If the only instruction required was 'Take this pill 30 minutes before bedtime,' matters would be greatly simplified, and much less demanding for all concerned.

Do I need to stop?

I think a lot of people go to their doctor worried that, one of these days, he or she is going to refuse to prescribe any more sleeping pills. Certainly I can think of patients who have felt that they were in the 'last-chance saloon'! They may have been told that they can have pills for one more month only, or have been advised to 'make them last'. Patients commonly recognize that they have gone the full circle with medication, and have not found anything that really solves the problem. Yet, the prospect of stopping may be very daunting.

All of this just reflects reality. The truth is that pharmacological solutions to persistent insomnia are not available. Doctors are under quite a bit of pressure not to prescribe treatments unless they are known to be effective, or unless they are clearly benefiting the individual patient. This can lead to quite a bit of momentum from the doctor's side to encourage you to stop. Of course, stopping is important to patients, too ... and may well be part of your goal in following this CBT program. Indeed, often patients say to me that they would feel much better about themselves if they could get off their medication. It is a goal in its own right. So my answer to the question 'Do I need to stop?' would be to take the bull by the horns. Go along to your doctor and have an honest discussion about your use of sleep medications. Discuss the specific medication that you are taking and about the length of time you have been on it. Discuss the potential benefits of staying on the pills relative to the benefits, and the difficulties, of withdrawing. Discuss whether or not there are any other pharmacological options. I am sure you would have your doctor's respect for doing this. I think decisions about medication should always be a *partnership* between patient and doctor. Ask your doctor if you can agree a joint plan, based upon what would be best for your health. That plan might well be a reduction schedule. You should also explain that you are following a structured CBT program, and describe a bit about the content of the program.

Can I take sleeping pills and use CBT?

Again this is a question that my patients raise. So, we should also consider the possibility that there may be some benefit associated with taking sleep medication as well as following the CBT program. This too is something you could discuss with your doctor.

After all, if medication affords some short-term benefit to sleep, and CBT is effective in the long term, would it not be possible to capitalize on a combined sleeping pill-plus-CBT approach? In many ways this is an attractive idea. It is also a very important research question, because in practice this combination is probably quite common. Unfortunately, however, we do not have enough data to give us a good answer to the question.

Only a couple of studies have been published on this so far. Results from this research reinforce the *importance of the CBT component* if people with insomnia are to obtain lasting benefit. As far as I can see from my reading there is no clear advantage for combining CBT with sleeping pills, except possibly in the first few weeks. There are also a couple of potential problems to look out for. One is that taking sleeping pills may reduce your attention to the CBT program, because taking pills is relatively easy by comparison. Another is that attributional problems can arise with combination therapies. You can never be sure what is causing any benefit that you experience. For example, you could (incorrectly) attribute treatment effects to the medication and so slacken off or even abandon some of the CBT methods. This would be likely to lead to a poor outcome because, of the two, CBT is the proven treatment. It could also lead in extreme cases to the development of dependency on medication.

How can I come off pills safely?

If you have decided that you want to stop taking sleeping pills, then you must consult your doctor. However, I can provide you with some general guidelines on good practice for safe withdrawal.

Over a period of time of taking medication for sleep, your body becomes used to the drug's chemical properties and to the concentration levels of the drug in your bloodstream. This process is known as *tolerance.* It is because of the build-up of tolerance that you may have experienced having to take a higher dose of your sleep medication in order to get the same effect. The fact that your body may have become used to the medication is one reason why a *gradual reduction* is essential.

Of course, the concentration of a drug in our bloodstream is something that is constantly changing as our bodies metabolize (use up) the chemical components of the drug. Different drugs are metabolized at different rates, and to give an indication of the length of time it takes our bodies to clear a compound, we use the term *half-life.* Half-life is the time (in hours) it takes for components of the drug to reduce their concentration by 50 per cent. So-called 'short-acting' drugs reach their peak concentrations in the bloodstream quickly and are eliminated quickly, whereas 'long-acting' drugs are usually slower to act, but also take much longer to clear. I have provided in Table 11.1 some information about the most commonly used sleep medications and their properties. I have given the generic names for the drug compounds in the table. It may be that you are prescribed medication under this name; alternatively, you may have one of these medications under a trade or brand name. These trade names differ from country to country, so you should check on the bottle or pill box to find the generic name of your medication on the list.

TABLE 11.1: SOME COMMONLY PRESCRIBED SLEEPING PILLS AND THEIR PROPERTIES

Sleeping pill (generic name)
Clonazepam
Normal dosage range (mg)
0.5–2
Half-life (hours)
20–60
Sleeping pill (generic name)
Estazolam
Normal dosage range (mg)
1–2
Half-life (hours)
8–24
Sleeping pill (generic name)
Flurazepam

Normal dosage range (mg)
15–30
Half-life (hours)
48–100
Sleeping pill (generic name)
Lorazepam
Normal dosage range (mg)
0.5–2
Half-life (hours)
10– 20
Sleeping pill (generic name)
Nitrazepam
Normal dosage range (mg)
5–10
Half-life (hours)
16–18
Sleeping pill (generic name)
Oxazepam
Normal dosage range (mg)
10–30
Half-life (hours)
5–10
Sleeping pill (generic name)
Quazepam
Normal dosage range (mg)
7.5–30
Half-life (hours)
40–120
Sleeping pill (generic name)
Temazepam
Normal dosage range (mg)

7.5–30
Half-life (hours)
8–17
Sleeping pill (generic name)
Triazolam
Normal dosage range (mg)
0.125–0.25
Half-life (hours)
2–4
Sleeping pill (generic name)
Zaleplon
Normal dosage range (mg)
5–10
Half-life (hours)
1
Sleeping pill (generic name)
Zolpidem
Normal dosage range (mg)
5–10
Half-life (hours)
1.5–5
Sleeping pill (generic name)
Zopiclone
Normal dosage range (mg)
3.75–7.5
Half-life (hours)
4–6

The advantage of short-acting sleeping pills is that, being more rapidly eliminated from the body, they tend to have fewer *carry-over effects* into the next day. By comparison, long-acting sleeping pills can lead to carry-over morning drowsiness. Clearly such effects are unwanted and can be dangerous, posing for example the risk of accidents. Although short-acting drugs avoid this particular problem, they are on the other hand more prone to *withdrawal effects,* because of their rapid elimination from the blood chemistry. Longer-acting drugs are eliminated more slowly and have a less abrupt withdrawal profile. As you will see in Table 11.1 there are some sleeping pills which are 'medium' in their effects, which means that they may either offer the best of both worlds, or possibly some degree of problem in both respects! The main advantage afforded by the newer nonbenzodiazepine hypnotics (those starting with the letter 'Z') is that they have been found to have fewer adverse effects upon the structure of sleep. That is, people may get a more natural sleep. They may also have a less severe withdrawal profile.

No doubt you will have heard people talking about having a 'fast metabolism' or a 'slow metabolism'. This reflects another important consideration. Medication should be prescribed and withdrawn *on an individual basis.* As a general rule, for example, older adults metabolize drugs more slowly and eliminate them more slowly, which means that older adults on certain medications are more likely to experience carry-over effects.

So I would stress that there is no absolute recommended withdrawal rate if you are planning to try to do without sleeping pills. You really need to consult your doctor. What I have done, though, is provide you in Box 11.1 (opposite) with a few pointers concerning a medication reduction schedule. It is particularly important that any withdrawal process should follow a gradual *tapering off.*

Can CBT help me come off sleep medication?

Sometimes people want to know if they can replace their sleep medication with CBT. They want to be able to trust another method, and hope that CBT may provide them with that opportunity. I think that this is a realistic possibility, but you need to think through what is likely to be the most successful means to that end for you. There are basically three options. All this is assuming you are following a gradual tapering off under medical supervision.

BOX 11.1 GENERAL ADVICE ON SLEEPING PILL WITHDRAWAL

1 Always consult your doctor when you are considering reducing or stopping sleep medication.

2 Obtain advice on a planned withdrawal schedule that suits your individual requirements. A suitable plan may require weeks or even months to complete. Typically you can expect to withdraw over an 8- to 10-week period.

3 Always reduce sleep medication by gradual tapering. Usually, small reductions in the medication dosage, or in the frequency of doses, will be advised by your doctor. Commonly reductions will be of around 25 per cent of the dosage, at intervals of one to two weeks.

4 Do not take additional medications or substitute medications unless they have been prescribed for you.

5 Tapering schedules should be reviewed weekly, or more frequently if you experience severe withdrawal effects.

6 Once you get down to the lowest prescribed dosage for each night, your doctor may recommend having 'drug holidays'. This is where you skip nights from taking this lowest dose, gradually skipping more and more nights until you stop altogether.

7 Keep a careful note (in your Sleep Diary and notebook) of your medication use, sleep pattern, and experiences associated with the withdrawal period.

8 Staying off sleeping pills can be difficult. Try to prevent relapse by identifying situations

coming up that might tempt you to take medication, and use CBT instead.

The first option is to withdraw medication gradually before commencing CBT. I will call this the 'withdraw-before' method. The main advantage here is that you can see what your underlying sleep pattern is like before starting CBT. As long as you have finally come off your sleeping pills for a few weeks, the withdraw-before option allows you to get a proper baseline on your sleep. It may even be that you won't have to start CBT if your sleep improves spontaneously once the medication is withdrawn. This does happen in some cases. The disadvantage, of course, is that it may not be easy to discontinue sleeping pills without some other strategy already in place.

The second option would be the 'withdraw-after ' method. The advantage here is that you don't need to start with the challenge of doing without pills and can concentrate straight away on the CBT program. If you see that your sleep is improving then you may gain sufficient confidence in CBT to enable you to withdraw. The disadvantage, though, is that your sleep pattern is likely to get disrupted again once the withdrawal process begins, and this might be difficult to deal with if you have only recently begun to sleep better. You should not expect that using CBT will mean that you can bypass drug-withdrawal effects, although it may help you cope with them better.

The third option is the 'withdraw-during' method. This might seem like the best compromise. However, you should bear in mind the disadvantage that it may be quite difficult to figure out how changes in your sleep pattern relate to the two things (CBT, withdrawal) that are going on at the same time.

How do you choose between these options? My advice would be to follow the one you are most likely to be able to carry through in practice. In other words, be *pragmatic* about this. The most important thing is to be able to take advantage of what CBT can offer and to stop medication if it is not benefiting you. If you can withdraw before and let the effects wash out of your system first, then that is probably ideal, but as I said – be pragmatic about what you are likely to be able to achieve … and good luck!

12

Recognizing and managing other common sleep disorders

Introduction

At various points throughout this book I have mentioned the importance of checking that you *do* have insomnia ... and checking that you *do not* have a different type of sleep problem. It is also possible that you could have more than one sleep disorder, of course.

In Chapter 3 I introduced you to the sleep disorders, and in Chapter 5 I gave you some tools to help you assess your sleep pattern and sleep symptoms. Remember I spoke about 'screening' procedures? Well, let me now introduce another bit of jargon that we use in clinical practice.

Clinicians are trained in what is known as *differential diagnosis.* That is the skill of distinguishing one type of disorder from another. When you are unwell you usually seek advice at first from a general medical practitioner, who begins the process of differential diagnosis. If it is thought that you need more specialized investigation or assessment, you may be referred on to someone else for an opinion. These days, diagnostic and treatment skills are becoming increasingly specialized, in every area of medicine. Sleep is no exception, and we now have clinicians who are sleep specialists. Often these doctors are neurologists or pulmonologists (respiratory specialists). The specialization in insomnia management has become known as *behavioral sleep medicine* and most professionals in this area are clinical psychologists.

I am not suggesting that you should do your own differential diagnosis. On the other hand, I think it is very helpful for you to be well informed about the key symptoms of different types of sleep disorder, so that if you do need to consult a professional you can have a more informed discussion about things. In particular, this chapter should help raise your awareness about five different groups of sleep disorders which may need managing in different ways. If you think that any of these might apply to you, you should make an appointment to see your doctor.

Aim

The aim of this chapter, therefore, is *to assist you in considering the possibility that you may have a sleep disorder other than insomnia, and to take steps to seek appropriate help.*

Disorders of the body clock (circadian disorders)

I am going to say a bit more about circadian disorders of sleep than about the other categories which follow because these disorders are more commonly confused with insomnia. You will see in Table 12.1 that I have provided you with a list of all the sleep disorders that we need to try to rule out.

We learned earlier that some body-clock functions are age-related. For example, the sleep drive of young adults can remain strong at 7a.m., compared to older adults where it begins to decline from about 5a.m. Later life is also associated with increases in sleepiness in the middle part of the evening. Another factor may simply be individual differences. Some people, regardless of age, have always tended to be 'larks' and others have tended to be 'owls'. So it is important that you consider both your age and your typical sleep time preferences before concluding that you have a circadian sleep disorder. In Table 12.1 there are two sub-categories of circadian problem that I want to mention. Let's take each of these in turn.

Delayed sleep phase syndrome (DSPS) often develops at a young age. You may not be surprised when you consider the key symptoms. This circadian disorder may present as a sleep-onset insomnia – that is, difficulty getting off to sleep. Central to the complaint is an inability to get to sleep at the desired time ... but there is also an inability to wake up at the desired time. In other words, the person with DSPS is out of step with the world by falling asleep late and waking and rising late. You might say 'typical of a teenager', but for the person with DSPS disorder this has not just been a temporary stage of growing up. Another feature is that there is usually little night-to-night variability in sleep pattern. The person with DSPS can, if left to their own schedule, have a normal sleep of good quality. They will fall asleep quickly (late on), sleep right through, and also 'sleep in'! Nevertheless, the EEG sleep stage distribution of their sleep will be normal. Typically, if they try to get up at a more normal hour (say 7a.m.) they will remain drowsy for some hours until their body clock reaches its wake time.

Another reason why DSPS might develop, and this also applies to other circadian problems, is when people have been *working shifts* and then try to get back into an 11p.m.-to-7a.m. sleep pattern. Usually people begin to adjust after a couple of weeks, but there are those who find this much harder. *Jet lag* is an even more common experience that is also usually temporary. Typically it takes anything from a few days to around ten days for your body clock to adjust to a different time zone. The bigger the time difference, the more adjustment needs to be made, of course. Nevertheless, it seems that people differ in their adaptability to these different types of circadian problem because adolescence, shiftwork, and international travel affect some people much more than others.

Advanced sleep phase syndrome (ASPS) is the opposite of DSPS. In ASPS problems are associated with early settling to bed and with early morning awakening. It is hard to 'keep going' during the evening because sleepiness kicks in early, and it is impossible to sustain sleep beyond 3 or 4a.m., or even earlier in extreme cases. ASPS is also the opposite of DSPS because it is more common in older people. Furthermore, the fragmentation of sleep in later life may lead to daytime napping, and this can contribute further to an already compromised circadian routine.

I should point out that of course our lifestyle plays a part in determining circadian disorders of the DSPS and ASPS variety. I have already mentioned the 'enforced' lifestyle of shiftwork. *Lifestyle choices* may also be implicated in the development of sleep phase disorders. For example, retired people may choose to retire early to bed because their lifestyle does not necessitate staying up late for a whole variety of reasons. In psychology we talk of *zeitgeber*s or 'time-givers'. These are the factors that determine the social rhythm of our lives – our routine. Developmental, social, and personal factors may all be zeitgebers. However, where sleep and wakefulness are concerned, natural light is the biggest zeitgeber of all. Generally speaking, we sleep when it is dark and we are awake in the daylight.

How can you know if you have circadian disorder rather than insomnia? Well, first of all consult the key symptom checklist in Table 12.1 overleaf. Also go back over the relevant part of the sleep history I gave you in Table 5.1. Another thing you can do is to look through your Sleep Diaries. I suggest taking at least two consecutive weeks, and longer if you can. Do you find that you tend to go to bed early and to wake early? Do you sleep well if you allow yourself to follow that routine? If so, ASPS is worth considering. Do you find that you don't properly wake up until hours after you rise in the morning? Do you find that you never get to sleep until the 'small hours'? If so then you could have DSPS.

TABLE 12.1: SLEEP DISORDERS OTHER THAN INSOMNIA: SUMMARY OF SYMPTOMS

Types of sleep disorder

Circadian disorder
Symptoms
Delayed sleep phase syndrome – awake till late, difficulty initiating sleep, difficulty walking in morning, still sleepy if rising at normal rising time, sleep normally if you go to bed very late and rise very late

Advanced sleep phase syndrome – evening sleepiness, difficulty delaying sleep till normal bedtime, early morning wakening, sleep normally if you go to bed very early and rise very early
Types of sleep disorder
Sleep-related breathing disorder
Symptoms
Obstructive sleep apnea – loud snoring (in most cases), breathing pauses, fragmented sleep with micro-arousals, daytime sleepiness, sometimes flat/depressed, often overweight
Types of sleep disorder
Restless legs and limb
Symptoms
Periodic limb movement disorder – involuntary jerky movements interrupting sleep, movements in sleeprepetitive pattern of movements, may have daytime sleepiness
Restless legs syndrome – irresistible urge to move legs when at rest, causing arousals from sleep
Types of sleep disorder
Parasomnias

Symptoms

Sleepwalking – occurs during incomplete arousals from deep sleep, difficult to waken, usually amnesic for event

Sleeptalking – normally occurs during transitions between sleep stages

Night terrors – often sit up in bed, strong emotional display, difficult to comfort or waken, usually amnesic for event

Confusional arousals – similar to sleepwalking, confused after wakening

Nightmares – emotionally laden dream content, often waken frightened from REM sleep

Teeth-grindmg (nocturnal bruxism) – occurs in different stages of sleep and at transitions

REM behavior disorder – muscle tone retained during REM sleep, dream enactment often aggressive

Types of sleep disorder

Narcolepsy and hypersomnia

Symptoms

Full narcolepsy syndrome comprises:

Sleep attacks – sudden involuntary sleeps in the daytime

Hypersomnia – excessive sleepiness and extended sleeps

Cataplexy – sudden loss of muscle tone in major muscle groups, in response to emotion

Hypnagogic/hypnopompic hallucinations – dream-like hallucinations upon entering/leaving sleep

Sleep paralysis – inability to move voluntarily, especially when emerging from sleep

If you can get access to an actigraphic assessment of your sleep, this will help with diagnosis. An *actigraph* is a device worn like a wristwatch that measures body movement and stores the information in an internal microchip for computer analysis. Active and inactive periods across several weeks are then displayed graphically, and it is possible to see what times of the day and night the natural peaks and troughs in movement occur. If they are out of alignment with the normal sleep (inactive) and wake (active) cycles, then this might suggest that you have a circadian problem. We are moving here into specialized assessment, though. You can't expect to get this kind of help from your local doctor. I would suggest that if you suspect DSPS or ASPS, you should take this thought to your doctor and consider with him or her what to do next. There are several options that might be considered.

Sometimes just *rescheduling* your sleep strictly, and gradually shifting your bedtime and rising time, can be effective. The aim is to move steadily closer and closer to the normal bedtime hours. For example, let's suppose the problem is DSPS and you think that you are three hours out of line (getting sleepy at 2a.m. and remaining sleepy till around 10a.m.). You might start by sleeping 2–10a.m. for one week, then shift to 1:45–9:45a.m. in week two, then to 1:30–9:30a.m. during week three, and so on, until you get to your desired schedule. If you had ASPS, you would reschedule too, but in the opposite direction of course!

There is also some evidence that oral *melatonin* supplementation can improve sleep timing, so it may be useful for DSPS and ASPS. The regulations surrounding the availability of melatonin vary from country to country. For example, in the USA melatonin can be purchased over the counter as a food supplement. In the UK it is available only on special prescription. Generally speaking, melatonin would be taken some hours before bed in DSPS and in the morning in ASPS. You will recall that the brain produces melatonin at night. Taking melatonin as a pill may be one way of enhancing sleep during the normal clock phase. Clearly you should follow the advice given by the manufacturer, by your pharmacist and by your doctor.

Finally, there is some evidence that *bright light therapy* can be used to improve circadian rhythm. This is connected to the melatonin story because, as we learned before, bright light shuts down the brain's production of melatonin.

In DSPS, bright light in the morning can help to advance the major sleep period, and in ASPS, bright light in the evening can help to delay sleep. Light boxes are commercially available in stores and on the web. If you want to use one of these you should again take care to read the instructions and limitations carefully. The evidence seems to be that 10,000 lux for 30 minutes or lower levels for longer periods is required to have a therapeutic effect.

It may be possible to combine the use of rescheduling, melatonin, and light therapy. As with the diagnosis of DSPS or ASPS, the treatment of circadian disorders should be conducted under skilled supervision. Certainly consult your doctor and consider the possibility of referral to a specialized Sleep Disorders Clinic.

Sleep-related breathing disorders (SBD)

This term refers to a group of disorders that seriously disrupt the continuity of sleep through impaired breathing. In some countries this field is known as *respiratory* medicine, in others the term *pulmonary* medicine is used. Either way, the point is that when breathing is affected during sleep, the quality of sleep that a person gets is likely to be poorer.

The most obvious and common example that comes to mind is *snoring.* Many people snore. This does not mean that they necessarily have a clinical problem with their sleep. Snoring is simply the sound made by the passage of air across a restricted airway. During sleep there is a tendency for the airway to 'collapse' (get narrower) so there is more respiratory effort involved in drawing air through the nose. Of course air contains the *oxygen* that sustains life, so as long as the brain can tell that we are getting enough oxygen into the bloodstream there is no problem – except perhaps for our partner having to listen to the noise!

However, if there is not enough air getting through, the bloodstream becomes *deoxygenated* or *desaturated.* Fortunately, the brain 'reads' this situation and causes us to arouse from sleep towards wakefulness, so that more normal breathing can recommence. It is also possible for people who do not snore to have respiratory problems of this kind, but snoring, being overweight and having a thick-set neck (with a collar size of 17 inches or more) are all closely related to sleep-related breathing disorders. SBDs are present in 2 per cent of men between the ages of 30 and 65, and in 1 per cent of women of the same age.

There is increasing public awareness of an SBD known as *obstructive sleep apnea* (OSA). In OSA, the upper airway collapses primarily during Stages 1 and 2 of sleep – that is, the lighter forms of non-REM sleep. An apnea is a complete closure/blockage of the upper airway. Basically, breathing stops. Partial, or incomplete, closures may also occur; these are known as hypopneas. In OSA apneaic and hypopneaic events disrupt sleep by causing *micro-arousals.* These brief wakenings are enough to cause *sleep fragmentation* and to decrease periods of Stage 3 and 4 and REM sleep.

How would you know if you have an SBD? Well, your most obvious night-time symptom would be difficulty remaining asleep. You might even be conscious of a tendency to wake out of sleep catching your breath, or of a feeling that you had stopped breathing. Some people wake themselves up with the sudden re-starting of their breathing after an apnea. Also, speak to your partner, who may be more aware of your breathing pattern or your snoring, and may have witnessed these 'breathing pauses'. Sometimes people with OSA wake with a headache and a very dry mouth in the morning.

OSA is associated also with daytime symptoms. The most important of these is *excessive daytime sleepiness.* Here there may be an involuntary tendency to fall asleep when at rest, or even when undertaking activities. Problems with concentration and irritability are often reported in OSA, and sleepiness has been linked to an increased likelihood of road traffic and industrial accidents. This is not a disorder to be taken lightly, because you and others can be at risk due to sleepiness. SBDs have also been associated with an increased risk of medical disorders, particularly of the cardiovascular system.

Clinical diagnosis of an SBD can only be confirmed through PSG assessment. These assessments include not only the standard sleep set-up (EEG, EOG, EMG) but also measurement of respiration and of blood-oxygen saturation levels. Of course assessment would also include a detailed interview, and partners are often invited to attend, for the reasons mentioned above. If you suspect that you may have an SBD, you should consult your doctor. Certainly if you have daytime sleepiness problems there is a distinct possibility that your sleep at night needs some investigation. Your doctor will know where to refer you.

Regarding treatment, *positional advice* to maximize breathing and to prevent airway collapse, and *weight loss* may be beneficial. Some dental *prosthetic devices* are also available. These are normally 'made to measure' and are worn in the mouth to improve breathing during sleep. Most of these devices serve to advance the lower jaw and extend the airway. *Surgery* is also used in some severe cases of OSA to rectify problems more permanently. At the symptomatic level, some *medications* that stimulate arousal and reduce daytime sleepiness may also help more mild to moderate cases.

The mainstay of treatment for OSA, however, is known as *continuous positive airway pressure* (CPAP). This is a simple mechanical pump which delivers a steady stream of air during sleep. This air is delivered under sufficient pressure to support the upper airway and to preventing collapse. Unfortunately, CPAP is not an elegant treatment. The most common clinical practice is to recommend use of a special mask that fits over the nose and is held in place by headgear consisting of straps. The mask is connected to a flexible tube through which air is delivered from the pump machine.

The good news is that CPAP is very effective at eliminating breathing pauses. This restores the natural pattern of sleep without interruption, and daytime symptoms reduce markedly. Normally people need to keep on using their CPAP machine long term if they want to stay symptom free.

Restless legs and limb movements in sleep

Periodic limb movement disorder (PLMD) and *restless legs syndrome* (RLS) are disorders that may occur in people who have SBD, or may exist even where there are no breathing disorders. Again there are no psychological treatments for PLMD or RLS; both conditions require careful assessment.

PLMD is mainly associated with older age, and involves muscle twitches in the limbs, particularly the legs, during sleep. These episodes of involuntary movement disrupt sleep, causing arousals from sleep Stages 1 and 2, leading to complaints of daytime sleepiness and insomnia. The diagnosis of PLMD must be confirmed by PSG showing that jerky leg movements are directly related to brief sleep arousals.

Most people have experienced the occasional involuntary limb movement. For example, many people get what we call *hypnic jerks* or *sleep starts* from time to time. These are sudden, brief jerky movements that occur at or around sleep-onset and wake us from light sleep. Hypnic jerks sometimes become a problem in their own right, but for most people they happen rarely. In some ways the movements in PLMD are similar to this, except they occur repeatedly and throughout the night.

We do not know exactly why people get PLMD. It may be related to disturbance of circadian sleep–wake rhythms in later life or to specific disorders of motor function that, again, occur more commonly in older adults. However, there are some medications that help PLMD. The options are either sedative-type drugs of the benzodiazepine family that reduce muscle function during sleep, or dopaminergic agents that are used to treat neuromuscular disorders.

RLS, as the name suggests, involves periods of irresistible urges to move the legs. These episodes are associated with unpleasant cramping sensations in the legs that are relieved only by walking or other movement or exercising of the legs. The symptoms begin mostly in the evening, potentially delaying the onset of sleep. So, they may occur when a person is resting or relaxing, and not only during sleep itself. When they interfere with sleep the usual result is sleep fragmentation and arousals. However, the relationship between RLS and daytime sleepiness is not clearly established. Normally people with RLS are able to give a clear picture of their problem, and they may have had it a long time. Although many people with RLS are of middle-age or older, about one-third of cases have their first symptoms before the age of 20.

The background to RLS is also a bit of a mystery, but like PLMD there may be associated changes in dopamine neurotransmissio n. Some of these may be age-related. RLS has also been associated with pregnancy and with end-stage renal (kidney) disease. Treatment of RLS is similar to that for PLMD, and indeed the two commonly go together. Some people with RLS are also given iron supplements.

Sleepwalking, night terrors, and other parasomnias

The *parasomnias* are a group of disorders that intrude into the sleep process and create disruptive behavioral events. They are associated with disorders of arousal, of partial arousal, or of transitions between different stages of sleep. Non-REM parasomnias are quite common during childhood, and in most instances resolve quite naturally. However, they can also persist into adulthood or, less commonly, begin then for the first time. The most common presentations of parasomnia include *sleepwalking (somnambulism), sleeptalking (somniloquy), night terrors* (sometimes called *sleep terrors),* and disorientation or confusion upon wakening *(confusional arousals).* These constitute primary parasomnias, and are disorders of arousal.

Other primary parasomnias include REM sleep disorders, such as *REM behavior disorder* (RBD). This is characterized by an absence of the muscle atonia that is normally present during REM sleep. In other words, someone with RBD may have retained motor function during dreaming sleep. So the person with RBD may be able to act out their dreams, carrying out complex and seemingly purposeful behavior while remaining physiologically asleep. Consequently, primary parasomnias and their associated behaviors – particularly sleepwalking and dream enactment – may lead to personal injury or injury to a bed partner. On rare occasions people have been known to carry out relatively complex tasks, like driving a car, during a parasomnia episode.

Precisely when these events occur during the night is often crucial in determining the underlying sleep disorder. For example, night terrors occur in Stage 3 or 4 sleep, often towards the end of the first or second phase of deep sleep. Therefore, like sleepwalking, they occur more commonly during the first third of the night. Because incomplete arousals out of deep sleep are involved, people who sleepwalk or have night terrors rarely have any accurate recall of what they were doing or what was on their mind at the time. This may seem surprising to the observer because the sleepwalker may appear purposeful in their activity, perhaps even trying to get out of the house or to find something. Similarly, a night terror is very distressing to watch because the person experiencing it appears extremely emotional and in a state of high physiological arousal and agitation. It is because the arousal is not a complete one and because the stage of sleep is a deep one that there is no conscious memory trace. Even if you do wake a sleepwalker or rouse someone from a night terror, they tend to remain 'groggy' and have only fleeting images or emotional statements to report.

By contrast, *nightmares* occur during REM sleep, which is, as we have learned, a relatively light form of sleep. They also relate more to the second half of the night, when REM episodes are more prolonged. These events often end with the dreamer actually waking up, so the memory trace is laid down more vividly. Indeed, because nightmares usually involve frightening or bizarre images, arousal from sleep is not only abrupt but lucid, and the person is unable to get back to sleep easily. Experts use the term *narrative recall* to describe the sleeper's ability to recount the occurrence and content of these dream events. The storyline is retained, and can sometimes be recurrent.

Having a better understanding of what is going on is the best treatment for all the parasomnias. *Information, education,* and *reassurance* are very important. Indeed, I quite often find that once I have explained the symptoms and given the diagnosis, patients with these problems may not need to come back to the clinic. We usually discover that there is an early history of, say, being prone to sleepwalking, and that some current stress factor has brought about a recurrence. Sometimes, though, people haven't acknowledged that they are under a strain – so be warned! On occasions I say to people that their parasomnia is 'like a friend tapping them on the shoulder and asking if they are sure they are OK'. So if you are the kind of person who copes with things very well on the surface, but tend to bury things you don't like to face, or if you bottle them up – then you will know I am speaking to you. Examining your individual *coping style* can be useful here.

Other things can make parasomnias more of a problem. *Sleep deprivation* is to be avoided, because if you are not getting enough sleep, the homeostatic pressure for sleep builds up. Too many late nights, particularly when accompanied by a change in life circumstances, can be fertile ground for parasomnias to arise. You see, in these circumstances your deep sleep and your REM sleep, the two most important sleep types, can go into 'rebound' – that is, you need more of them as your body tries to catch up on lost sleep. Consequently the likelihood of parasomnia increases because you spend more time in the sleep states that play host to parasomnia problems.

A related risk factor is *alcohol,* because alcohol also plays around with the natural proportions of our night's sleep. You can certainly be more prone to parasomnias after drinking, so I advise people who have problems with parasomnias to drink in very careful moderation, if at all. You will realize, too, that these risk factors can converge when you are staying up late, drinking, out of your usual routines and trying to deal with stressful problems all at once.

I also want to mention *safety* and what might be called *risk assessment.* If you get out of bed and you are not properly awake, then you are potentially at greater risk of injury. I mentioned before that some sleepwalkers try to go outdoors, even through windows. Some people can be more likely to sleepwalk in unfamiliar places, which of course carries its own risks. It is important, therefore, that you consider potential risk factors and address these with your family or the people you live with.

Before leaving this section I want to return briefly to RBD. This is most common in middle-aged or older men. It can occur on its own, or it can be associated with motor disorders that occur mainly later on in life, such as Parkinson's disease. It can also be caused or made worse by some medications. So these things should be checked out with your doctor. In RBD it is quite common for a bed partner to get injured during the enactment of the sleeper's dreams, and this is the most frequent trigger to help-seeking, in my experience. Once again, all the components of management that I have already mentioned are important with RBD, plus a diagnostic PSG assessment if you and your doctor feel that this is necessary. There are some drugs that can help reduce or eliminate the symptoms of RBD.

Narcolepsy and hypersomnia

There are a number of key characteristic symptoms associated with *narcolepsy.* Some of these relate to the sleep period and some to daytime. *Hypersomnia* is a term we use for excessive sleepiness, and it can occur without all the symptoms of the full narcolepsy syndrome.

Narcolepsy causes extreme daytime sleepiness, which can lead to a *sleep attack.* Normally we fall asleep gradually and we notice the increasing signs of drowsiness along the way. People with narcolepsy can sometimes be aware of their sleepiness, which is very extreme, but they also have sudden sleep attacks that come on more or less out of the blue. Another daytime symptom is called *cataplexy.* This can also occur very suddenly in the form of a cataplectic attack when the body muscles give way, often triggered by extremes of emotion such as humour or anger.

At night, narcolepsy is associated with abnormalities of REM sleep. *Hypnagogic hallucinations* are vivid, dreamlike experiences that occur around sleep-onset, and *hypnopompic hallucinations* are similar phenomena that arise in the morning upon waking. People with narcolepsy go into REM sleep quite readily and so they can experience these transitional dream experiences as if they were part of normal consciousness.

There is another unusual symptom known as *sleep paralysis.* This is a period of inability to perform voluntary movements either at sleep-onset or upon waking. In simple terms, the mind wakes up but the body remains paralysed. So you will see that narcolepsy is a strange disorder with a number of quite frightening symptoms.

In recent years genetic markers for this disorder have been identified, and this has improved the accuracy of narcolepsy diagnoses. Diagnosis can only be fully determined, however, through full PSG assessment and a procedure known as a *multiple sleep latency test* (MSLT). The MSLT involves attending a sleep laboratory and being given successive 'sleep opportunities' across a period of time. The goal is to detect how rapidly sleep occurs, and to explore the sleep-stage characteristics of the sleep that is observed. The possibility of *rapid-onset REM sleep* is one of the features that is being investigated in an MSLT, because this is common in narcolepsy but rare in normal sleepers.

Effective pharmacological treatments have been developed for narcolepsy. These are mostly *stimulant drugs* to help sustain wakeful brain function. Although these drugs are effective, they treat only the symptoms. Addressing *behavioral factors* such as maintaining a stable sleep pattern, avoiding sleep deprivation, and taking scheduled daytime naps also helps.

Further help

We started in Part Two with the idea of screening for the possibility that you may have a sleep problem other than insomnia. You have now read this additional chapter to help you to clarify that possibility. I hope that you are now a bit further on in your own thinking on the matter. Your next step should be to make an appointment to see your doctor. Take your new found knowledge, your thoughts, and concerns with you to that appointment. You can then discuss the possibility of referral to a specialist sleep clinic if that seems to be the best way forward.

Glossary

actigraph a simple device, usually worn on the wrist, that measures body movement and provides an estimate of time spent awake and time spent asleep.

advanced sleep phase syndrome (ASPS) a circadian disorder of sleep where the 'body clock' is set to fall asleep early and to wake early.

attention bias a tendency to selectively focus, to find your attention drawn to something. In the case of insomnia the focus is upon sleep and wakefulness.

attention–intention–effort an insomnia process where attention bias leads to intentional sleep and then to effortful sleep, all of which cause wakefulness.

attributions the beliefs that people hold about the causes of a problem.

automaticity the natural and involuntary process of sleep in good sleepers. This is disrupted by attention–intention–effort in insomnia.

circadian rhythm the regular sleep–wake cycle that is determined by a 'body clock' mechanism in the brain.

delayed sleep phase syndrome (DSPS) a circadian disorder of sleep where the body clock is set to fall asleep late and to wake late.

Diagnostic and Statistical Manual of Mental Disorders (DSM) a schedule used by mental health professionals to diagnose mental health problems.

electroencephalography (EEG) the measurement of electrical activity in the brain from scalp electrodes.

electromyography (EMG) the measurement of muscle activity using electrodes attached to the body (commonly to the chin and legs).

electro-oculography (EOG) the measurement of eye movements using electrodes attached at the side of the eye sockets.

hypnogram a graphical presentation of sleep showing transitions between sleep stages in fine detail across the night.

International Classification of Sleep Disorders (ICSD) a schedule used by sleep experts to diagnose different sleep disorders.

melatonin a naturally occurring brain hormone that helps to regulate circadian rhythm.

multiple sleep latency test (MSLT) a test of daytime sleepiness that indicates how sleep deprived a person is.

narcolepsy a sleep disorder characterized by excessive sleepiness, sleep attacks, and a number of specific features.

non-REM sleep sleep stages 1, 2, 3 and 4 form 75 per cent of the night's sleep, with Stage 2 being the most common.

obstructive sleep apnea a sleep-related breathing disorder involving breathing pauses during sleep that make people excessively sleepy during the daytime.

paradoxical insomnia a complaint of insomnia whereby people feel that they hardly ever sleep at all; formerly known as sleep-state misperception.

parasomnias a group of sleep disorders characterized by nocturnal activity during partial arousals from sleep or transitions between sleep stages. The most common non-REM parasomnias are sleepwalking, sleeptalking, and night terrors. The most common REM parasomnias are nightmares.

periodic limb movement disorder (PLMD) periodic limb movements during sleep involving repetitive jerky movements. They can constitute a disorder when they disrupt sleep.

polysomnography (PSG) the detailed measurement of the sleep process using many (poly) measurements including EEG, EMG and EOG. PSGs are usually conducted in a lab, but there are portable systems for home use.

primary insomnia a primary insomnia is a disorder of sleep in its own right, not caused by some other known factor such as a medical condition.

psychophysiologic insomnia a primary insomnia caused largely by psychological factors including conditioned arousal in bed and sleep-related worry. See also attention–intention–effort.

randomized controlled trial (RCT) a scientific study that tests the effectiveness of a treatment under controlled conditions, taking account of chance and often also of placebo factors.

rapid eye movement sleep (REM sleep) periods of sleep when the body is very still but the brain is very active (often dreaming). Named after its characteristic eye movements.

rebound insomnia an insomnia caused by withdrawal effects from drugs of a sedative nature.

restless legs syndrome (RLS) a sleep disorder characterized by unpleasant sensations in the legs, relieved only by movement.

secondary insomnia an insomnia associated with, or caused by, a medical or psychiatric disorder.

sleep deprivation the consequences of insufficient sleep involving fatigue, daytime sleepiness, and increased drive for recovery sleep.

sleep efficiency (SE) the proportion of time in bed that is spent asleep, expressed as a percentage.

sleep homeostasis the drive for sleep that is governed primarily by the amount of time spent awake. The homeostat tries to create a balance by satisfying sleep needs.

sleep-onset latency (SOL) time taken to fall asleep after going to bed and putting out the light.

sleep stages sleep is divided into different stages (non-REM stages 1 to 4, REM sleep, wake and movement time) using standard scoring criteria.

sleep-state misperception former term for paradoxical insomnia.

time in bed (TIB) the period from retiring to rising.

total sleep time (TST) hours and minutes of sleep on a given night.

total wake time (TWT) the total of SOL plus WASO.

wake time after sleep-onset (WASO) the total time spent awake during night-time awakenings (after first falling asleep).

Useful organizations

For information on psychotherapies and CBT
Association for Behavioral and Cognitive Therapies (ABCT)
305 Seventh Avenue 16th Floor
New York, NY 10001-6008
USA
Tel: (001)212-647-1890
Fax: (001)212-647-1865
Web site: www.aabt.org

British Association for Behavioural and Cognitive Psychotherapies (BABCP)
Victoria Buildings
9–13 Silver Street
Bury
BL9 0EU
Tel: 0161-797-4484
Fax: 0161-797-2670
Email: babcp@babcp.com
Web site: www.babcp.com

European Association for Behavioural and Cognitive Therapies (EABCT)
EABCT Office
Maliebaan 50B
3581 CS Utrecht
The Netherlands

Tel: 00-31-30-254-3054
Fax: 00-31-30-254-3037
Email: eabct@vgct.nl
Web site: www.eabct.com

For information on insomnia and sleep problems:

American Academy of Sleep Medicine (AASM)

1 Westbrook Corporate Center, Suite 920
Westchester
Illinois 60154
USA
Tel: (001)708-492-0930
Fax: (001)708-492-0943
Email: inquires@aasmnet.org
Web site: www.aasmnet.org

Australasian Sleep Association (ASA)

GPO Box 295
Sydney
NSW 1043
Australia
Tel: (0061)0500-500-701
Fax: (0061)0500-500-702
Email: sleepaus@ozemail.com.au
Web site: www.sleepaus.on.net

British Sleep Society (BSS)

PO Box 247
Colne, Huntingdon
UK
PE28 3UZ
Email: enquiries@sleeping.org.uk
Web site: www.sleeping.org.uk

Canadian Sleep Society (CSS)
Hôpital du Sacré-Coeur de Montréal
Centre de Recherche, 3K
5400, boul. Gouin Ouest
Montréal
QC H4J 1C4
Canada
Email: info@css.to
Web site: www.css.to

European Sleep Research Society (ESRS)
Sleep Disorders Unit
Department of Neurology
Fundacíon Jiménez Diaz
Avda. de los Reyes Católicos, 2
28040 Madrid
Spain
Tel: (0034)91-543-1423 or (0034)91-550-4927
Fax: (0034)91-543-9316
Email: dgb@iis.es
Web site: www.esrs.org

National Sleep Foundation (NSF)
1522 K Street NW
Suite 500
Washington, DC 20005
USA
Tel.: (001)202-347-3471
Fax: (001)202-347-3472
Email: nsf@sleepfoundation.org
Web site: www.sleepfoundation.org

Further reading

Ancoli-Israel, Sonia, *All I Want is a Good Night's Sleep,* Mosby-Year Book, Inc.: St Louis, 1996

Cole, Frances, et al, *Overcoming Chronic Pain,* Constable & Robinson: London, 2010

Dement, William C. and Vaughan, Christopher C., *The Promise of Sleep: The Scientific Connection Between Health, Happiness and a Good Night's Sleep,* Macmillan: London, 2000

Gilbert, Paul, *Overcoming Depression,* Constable & Robinson: London, 2009

Kennerley, Helen, *Overcoming Anxiety,* Constable & Robinson: London, 2009

Lavie, Peretz, *The Enchanted World of Sleep,* Yale University Press: Newhaven and London, 1996

Morin, Charles M., *Relief from Insomnia: Getting the Sleep of Your Dreams,* Doubleday: New York, 1996

Morin, Charles M. and Espie, Colin A., *Insomnia: A Clinical Guide to Assessment and Treatment,* Kluwer Academic/Plenum Press: New York, 2003

Szuba, Martin P., Kloss, Jacqueline D. and Dinges, David F., *Insomnia: Principles and Management,* Cambridge University Press: Cambridge, 2003

More psychology titles from Constable & Robinson
Please visit www.overcoming.co.uk for more information

Title

An Introduction to Coping with Anxiety
An Introduction to Coping with Depression
An Introduction to Coping with Health Anxiety
An Introduction to Coping with Obsessive Compulsive Disorder
An Introduction to Coping with Panic
An Introduction to Coping with Phobias
Overcoming Anger and Irritability
Overcoming Anorexia Nervosa
Overcoming Anxiety
Overcoming Anxiety Self-Help Course (3 parts)
Overcoming Body Image Problems
Overcoming Bulimia Nervosa and Binge-Eating – new edition
Overcoming Bulimia Nervosa and Binge-Eating Self-Help Course (3 parts)
Overcoming Childhood Trauma
Overcoming Chronic Fatigue
Overcoming Chronic Pain
Overcoming Compulsive Gambling
Overcoming Depersonalizaton and Feelings of Unreality
Overcoming Depression – new edition

Overcoming Depression: Talks With Your Therapist (audio)

Overcoming Grief

Overcoming Health Anxiety

Overcoming Insomnia and Sleep Problems

Overcoming Low Self-Esteem

Overcoming Low Self-Esteem Self-Help Course (3 parts)

Overcoming Mood Swings

Overcoming Obsessive Compulsive Disorder

Overcoming Panic and Agoraphobia

Overcoming Panic and Agoraphobia Self-Help Course (3 parts)

Overcoming Paranoid and Suspicious Thoughts

Overcoming Problem Drinking

Overcoming Relationship Problems

Overcoming Sexual Problems

Overcoming Social Anxiety and Shyness

Overcoming Social Anxiety and Shyness Self-Help Course (3 parts)

Overcoming Stress

Overcoming Traumatic Stress

Overcoming Weight Problems

Overcoming Worry

Overcoming Your Child's Fears and Worries

Overcoming Your Child's Shyness and Social Anxiety

Overcoming Your Smoking Habit

The Compassionate Mind

The Happiness Trap

The Glass Half-Full
I Had a Black Dog
Living with a Black Dog
Manage Your Mood: How to use Behavioral
Activation Techniques to Overcome Depression
P&P

Name (block letters): _____
Address:_____
Postcode:_____
Email: Tel No:_____
How to Pay:

1. By telephone: call the TBS order line on 01206 255 800 and quote ESPIE. Phone lines are open between Monday–Friday, 8.30am–5.30pm.

2. By post: send a cheque for the full amount payable to TBS Ltd, and send form to: Freepost RLUL-SJGC-SGKJ. Cash Sales/Direct Mail Dept, The Book Service, Colchester Road, Frating, Colchester, CO7 7DW

Is/are the book(s) intended for personal use _ or professional use_?

Please note this information will not be passed on to third parties.

Back Cover Material

The Overcoming self-help guides use Cognitive Behavioral Therapy (CBT) techniques to treat disorders by changing unhelpful patterns of behavior and thought. CBT is internationally favoured as a practical means of overcoming long-standing and disabling conditions, both psychological and physical. Many guides in the Overcoming series are recommended by the UK Department of Health under the Books on Prescription scheme.

***

Poor sleep is one of the most common health problems, but prescribed medications and over-the-counter remedies rarely offer lasting benefits. Now research conducted over 25 years has established cognitive behavioral therapy as the treatment of choice for insomnia, and in this new guide, CBT principles have been incorporated into a complete course of self-help.

- **How to improve your sleeping environment**
- **Developing good pre-bedtime routines**
- **Learning to relax**
- **Establishing a new sleeping and waking pattern**
- **How to deal with a racing mind**

- **More effective use of sleeping pills**
- **Special problems including jet lag and sleepwalking**

PROFESSOR COLIN ESPIE is Professor of Clinical Psychology and Director of the University of Glasgow Sleep Centre. He is a leading member of the American Academy of Sleep Medicine and the British Sleep Society.

A

actigraph assessment, *315*

advanced sleep phase syndrome (ASPS), *315, 317, 318*
  in older people, *312*
alcohol, *113, 126, 145, 166, 169, 173, 272, 328*
American Academy of Sleep Medicine, *73, 197*
antidepressant drugs, *73*
  tricyclic, *73*
anxiety, *57, 60, 63, 155, 176, 256, 262*
Aserinsky, Dr, *13*
assessing your insomnia problem, *99, 100, 101, 103, 109, 113, 126, 127, 128, 130, 132, 134*
  see also Sleep Diary, goals for, *128, 130, 132*
  using a sleep diary, *109, 113, 126, 127, 128, 130, 132, 134*
  and your personal sleep history, *100, 101*

attentional bias, *66, 67, 260*
  see also insomnia, sleep-related, *66*
  threat-related, *67*
automaticity, *29, 39, 64, 67, 69, 70, 263*
as cause of insomnia, *156*

B

bed–sleep connection (and), *198, 200, 201, 203, 204*
  avoiding napping, *203, 204*
  see also napping,
bedtime activities, *200*
  feeling sleepy, *203*
  quarter-of-an-hour rule, *200, 201*
  evaluating, *263, 264*
body clock, *28, 45, 311*
  see also circadian disorders; circadian rhythm and circadian timer,
booster therapy, *288*
Bootzin, Dr Richard, *197*

boxes,
  calculating average sleep time, *208*
  different types of relaxation, *184*
  imagery training essentials, *252*
  overview of CBT program, *271, 272, 274*
  putting the day to rest, *247, 248*
  relaxation summary, *191*
  rising time, *210*
  sleep quiz, *139*
  sleep scheduling program summary, *216, 217*
  sleeping pill withdrawal, *305*
  thought-blocking, *248*
  threshold time, *211*
  tips on completing sleep diary, *127*
bright light therapy, *317, 318*

C

caffeine, *37, 166, 168, 169, 173, 269, 272*
children,
  sleep requirements of, *30, 37, 141*
  and tiredness, *81*
circadian disorders, *309, 311, 312, 315, 317, 318*
  actigraph assessment for, *315*
  advanced sleep phase syndrome (ASPS), *312, 315, 317, 318*
  bright light therapy for, *317*
  delayed sleep phase syndrome (DSPS), *311, 312, 315, 317, 318*
  jet lag, *311, 312*
  and lifestyle choices, *312*
circadian rhythm, *28, 29, 38, 62, 176, 317*
  and afternoon dip, *29*
circadian timer, *26, 29, 70*
clock-watching, *260, 262, 263*
coffee, *37, 165, 166, 168, 170, 269, 272*
  analysis of attributions, *83*
  behavioral sleep medicine, *73*

persistent insomnia, *73, 294*

see also insomnia, programs for insomnia, *57, 96*

see also individual subject entries, assessing your insomnia problem, *99, 100, 101, 103, 109, 113, 126, 127, 128, 130, 132, 134*

overview, *271, 272, 274*

'putting it all together', *266, 267, 269, 271, 272, 274, 276, 288*

racing mind, *221, 222, 223, 225, 227, 228, 229, 245, 247, 248, 250, 252, 253, 255, 256, 258, 260, 262, 263, 264*

sleep hygiene and relaxation, *165, 166, 168, 169, 170, 172, 173, 174, 176, 177, 179, 180, 181, 182, 184, 185, 187, 188, 189, 191, 192, 194, 195*

sleep pattern scheduling, *197, 198, 200, 201, 203, 204, 206, 208, 210, 211, 213, 214, 216, 217, 219*

understanding sleep and insomnia, *136, 137, 139, 141, 142, 144, 145, 147, 148,* *150, 151, 152, 154, 155, 156, 158, 159, 161, 163*

concentration, *54, 78, 79, 82, 85, 154, 288*

consequences of insomnia, *75, 76, 78, 79, 81, 82, 83, 85, 86, 88, 89, 90*

see also insomnia and sleep,

D

daytime tiredness, *139, 151*

dealing with a racing mind,

see racing mind, de-catastrophizing situations, *255*

deep sleep, *12, 13, 19, 22, 32, 35, 37, 141, 142, 150, 151, 169, 172, 325, 328*

definitions of sleep, *5, 6*

delta waves, *12, 151*

Dement, Dr William C., *26*

dependency problems, *71, 154, 299*

depression, *57, 71, 81, 82, 155, 227, 228*

Diagnostic and Statistical Manual of

Mental Disorders (DSM), *51, 54, 58*

diet, *166, 169, 170, 173*

differential diagnosis, *308, 309*

  and dream enactment, *325, 327*

drugs,

  see alcohol; caffeine; nicotine and sleeping pills,

E

earplugs and noise, *173, 174*

Edinger, Dr Jack, *20*

electroencephalography (EEG), *6, 7, 9, 12, 13, 15, 311, 321*

  channels, *19, 20*

  patterns, *151*

electromyography (EMG), *7, 9, 12, 13, 15, 321*

electro-oculography (EOG), *7, 9, 12, 13, 15, 321*

Enchanted World of Sleep, The, *5, 6*

  exercise, physical, *166, 170, 172, 173, 271*

  see also relaxation,

eye movements, *7*

  rapid, *13*

rolling, *12*

F

fatigue, *30, 37, 38, 60, 76, 78, 79, 85*

  daytime, *55*

figures,

  bedtime wind-down, *181*

  changes in sleep patterns across a life span, *36*

  commitment and unproductive effort, line between, *194*

  considering your motivational state, *132*

  Glasgow Content of Thoughts Inventory (GCTI), *229, 245*

  insomnia as common problem, *59*

  model of insomnia development, *64*

  predisposing, precipitating and perpetuating factors in insomnia, *62*

  sleep diary, *113*

sleep hygiene factors to improve sleep pattern, *180*

sleep hypnogram in childhood, young adulthood and later life, *32*

sleep laboratory assessment, *7*

stages of sleep: polysomnographic (PSG) recording, *9*

G

Glasgow Content of Thoughts Inventory GCTI), *228, 229, 245, 263*

Glasgow Sleep Effort Scale (GSES), *69, 70, 256, 258*

goal(s), *99, 128, 130, 132, 134*

achievable and measurable, *132, 271*

improvement, *276*

maintenance, *276*

H

health problems, *55, 57, 58, 86, 154, 294*

see also mental health problems and sleep disorders,

physical, *57*

respiratory, *55*

humour, *255, 330*

hypnagogic hallucinations, *330*

hypnogram, *19, 32, 35*

hypnopompic hallucinations, *330*

I

insomnia (and), *22, 23, 38, 39, 41, 43, 45, 51, 52, 54, 55, 57, 58, 59, 60, 62, 63, 64, 66, 67, 69, 70, 71, 73, 148, 152*

see also assessing your insomnia problem; napping and sleep, attention–intention–effort cycle, *29*

behavioral sleep medicine for, *73*

characteristics of, *51, 52, 54*

as chronic problem, *86, 88*

cognitive behavior therapy (CBT), *57, 73, 88, 89, 90*

see also main entry,

as common problem, *58, 59, 60, 62*

concentration problems, *78, 79, 82*

coping and everyday life, *82, 83*

depression, *81, 82, 86*

development from occasional to persistent, *62, 63, 64*

diagnosis of, *103*

diagnostic classification systems for, *51*

effect on family, *83, 85*

effect on social and working life, *85, 86*

effortful process for, *69, 70*

hypnotic-dependent, *57*

impact on experience of sleep, *75, 76*

insomnia development model, *64, 66, 67, 69, 70*

life changes, *155*

medication for, *70, 71, 73*

paradoxical, *25, 26, 55, 103*

perpetuating factors for, *63*

persistence of, *152, 294*

predispositions to, *62, 63*

psychophysiologic, *23, 54, 70, 103*

secondary, *55, 57, 103*

sleeping pills and rebound, *58, 71*

sub-types, *54, 55, 57, 58*

triggers for, *48, 49*

International Classification of Sleep Disorders (ICSD), *51, 54, 58*

irritability, *79, 81, 83, 139, 148, 150, 154, 253*

K

Kales, Dr, *15*

Kleitman, Dr, *13*

L

latency,
  and multiple sleep latency test (MSLT), *331*
  to REM onset, *19*
  sleep-onset (SOL), *18, 52*

Lavie, Peretz, *5, 6*

Lichstein, Dr Kenneth, *57*

life changes and insomnia, *155*

long and short sleepers, *46*

M

measuring sleep (by), *6, 7, 9*

  see also individual subject entries, electroencephalography (EEG), *6, 7, 321*

  electromyography (EMG), *7, 321*

  electro-oculography (EOG), *7, 321*

  polysomnography (PSG), *9*

medication, *58, 71, 321*

  see also sleeping pills, hypnotic drugs, *71*

  and older people, *303*

  over-the-counter remedies, *89*

  for PMLD, *328, 330*

  and randomized controlled trials (RCTs), *89*

  reduction schedules, *303*

melatonin, *28, 317, 318*

mental health problems, *57, 58, 103, 228*

  insomnia, fatigue and irritability, *79, 81*

  monitoring sleep, *219*

  see also Sleep Diary, Morin, Dr Charles, *63, 161*

motivation, wheel of, *288*

motivation for change, *132, 134, 194, 219*

movement time (M), *19, 20*

multiple sleep latency test (MSLT), *331*

music, listening to, *201*

muscle tone measurement, see electromyography (EMG),

N

napping, *37, 38, 154, 155, 312*

  avoiding, *28, 38, 203, 204*

narcolepsy, *151, 330, 331*

  behavioral factors in, *331*

  and hypersomnia, *330, 331*

neurological problems, *55*

nicotine, *166, 168, 169, 173*

normal sleep, *5, 6, 7, 9, 12, 13, 15, 18, 19, 20, 22, 23, 25, 26, 28, 29, 30*

   see also definitions and stages of sleep, normal variations in sleep, *32, 35, 36, 37, 38, 39, 41, 42, 43, 45, 46, 48, 49*

O

older people (and), *37, 48, 141*

   ASPS, *312*
   changes in sleep pattern, *35, 151, 309*
   napping, *38, 312*
   PLMD, *322*
oversleeping, *147*

P

Perlis, Dr Michael, *23*
phobias, *67, 136, 198*
pineal gland, *28*
polysomnography (PSG), *9, 20, 23, 25, 55, 321, 322, 330, 331*
poor sleep, *22, 30, 38, 39, 41*
   see also insomnia, triggers to, *48, 49*

pre-bedtime routine (and), *172, 173, 174, 176, 177, 179, 180, 181, 182*

   air quality, *176*
   body temperature, *174*
   dealing with noise, *172, 173, 174*
   lighting, *176*
   mattress and pillows, *177, 179*
   room temperature, *174*
   wind-down routine, *179, 180, 181, 182*
'putting it all together', *266, 267, 269, 271, 272, 274, 276, 288*
   with confident approach to program, *267, 269, 271, 272, 274*
   by making lasting changes, *288*
   by trusting evidence for CBT, *276*

R

racing mind (and), *221, 222, 223, 225, 227, 228, 229, 245, 247, 248, 250, 252, 253, 255, 256, 258, 260, 262, 263, 264*

   attention and clock-watching, *260, 262, 263*

common thought patterns,
see thoughts,
evaluating daytime feelings, *263, 264*
giving up trying to sleep, *253, 255, 256*
Glasgow Sleep Effort Scale (GSES), *256, 258, 260*
imagery, *252, 253*
relaxation as distraction technique, *250, 252, 253*
sleep scheduling, *253, 264*
rapid eye movement (REM) sleep, *13, 35, 37, 42, 145, 325, 327, 328, 330, 331*
behavior disorder (RBD) of, *325, 328, 330*
and non-REM sleep, *13, 37, 151*
rapid-onset, *331*
reading in bed, *200*
Rechtschaffen, Dr, *15*
record identification information, *15*
relapses, *134, 219*
prevention of, *288*

relaxation, *182, 184, 185, 187, 188, 189, 191*
active and passive, *182, 184*
and progressive relaxation training technique, *184, 185, 187, 188, 189, 191*
and summary of program, *191*
dysfunctional thinking (Morin), *161*
insomnia, *23, 221, 222*

S
sleep, *5, 6, 13, 26*
self-evaluation, *262, 263*
self-monitoring, *262*
sleep (and), assessment (PSG), *20, 22, 23, 25*
see also Sleep Diary,
attentional bias, *64, 66, 67, 253*
automaticity, *29, 66, 67, 69*
bad night's, *152*
circadian rhythm, *28*
circadian timer, *26*
deep,
see deep sleep,
deprivation, *42, 43, 328*

358

doing without, *156*
efficiency (SE), *18, 22, 288*
effort, *69, 70*
evaluative process, *69*
good sleepers, *191, 192*
homeostat, *26, 39*
inertia, *147*
length of adult sleep, *150*
melatonin, *28, 317*
memory, *145, 147*
need for, *29, 30*
non-restorative, *51*
parameters, *15*
perceptions of, *25, 26*
see also insomnia,
preoccupation with, *70, 258*
quality of, *22*
rapid eye movement,
see rapid eye
movement (REM)
sleep,
recovery, *35*
slow-wave, *12*
stage 1 of 8, *12*
synchronized, *13*
variations in,
see variations in
sleep,
sleep debt, *26, 28, 35, 43, 144*

see also napping,
Sleep Diary, *22, 99, 101, 150, 161, 163, 195, 206, 219, 264, 271, 274, 276, 315*
  for assessing
  insomnia, *109, 113, 126, 127, 128, 130, 132, 134, 276*
sleep disorders
breathing,
  see sleep-related,
  breathing disorder
  (SBD), *109, 318, 320, 321, 322*
  circadian (body
  clock), *309, 311, 312, 315, 317, 318*
  see also circadian
  disorders,
  narcolepsy and
  hypersomnia, *330, 331*
  nightmares, *327*
  parasomnias, *324, 325, 327, 328*
  periodic limb
  movement disorder
  (PLMD), *322, 324*
  recognizing and
  managing common,
  308, 309, 311, 312, 315, 317, 318, 320, 321, 322, 324, 325, 327, 328, 330, 331

REM behavior disorder (RBD), *325, 328, 330*

REMsleep behavior, *13, 325, 327*

restless legs syndrome (RLS), *322, 324*

  sleep paralysis, *331*

  sleepwalking, *13, 324, 325*

sleep efficiency (SE), *18, 22, 52*

sleep effort, *253, 256, 258*

sleep homeostat, *26*

sleep hygiene and relaxation, *165, 166, 168, 169, 170, 172, 173, 174, 176, 177, 179, 180, 181, 182, 184, 185, 187, 188, 189, 191, 192, 194, 195*

  see also relaxation and Sleep Diary, and good sleepers, *191, 192*

  lifestyle factors for, *166, 168, 169, 170, 172*

  see also alcohol; diet; drugs and exercise, pre-bedtime routine for, see pre-bedtime routine,

sleep laboratory, *6, 7, 9*

quality of sleep in, *20*

sleep loss, *43*

sleep-onset-latency (SOL), *18, 23, 52*

sleep maintenance (WASO), *18, 23, 52*

  and amount of sleep needed, *204, 206, 208*

  bed–sleep connection, *198, 200, 201, 203, 204*

  see also main entry, making adjustments in, *219*

  motivation, *217, 219*

  nightly schedule, *214, 216*

  setting time in bed with, *208, 210, 211, 213*

    rising time, *210*

    threshold time, *210, 211, 213*

  window, *213, 214, 219, 288*

sleep patterns, *35, 83, 288*

  age-related changes in, *35, 36, 37*

  optimizing, *263*

sleep-related breathing disorders (SBD), *109, 318, 320, 321, 322*

  clinical diagnosis of, *321*

obstructive sleep apnea (OSA), *320, 321, 322*
  and continuous positive airway pressure (CPAP), *321, 322*
  daytime symptoms of, *320, 321*
  prosthetic devices for, *321*
  snoring, *109, 318, 320*
sleep reports (and), *15, 18, 19, 20*
  see also stages of sleep,
  latency to REM onset, *19*
  movement time (M), *19, 20*
  record identification information, *15*
  sleep efficiency (SE), *18, 22, 52*
  sleep parameters, *15*
  sleep-onset-latency (SOL), *18, 23, 52*
  time in bed (TIB), *18*
  total sleep time (TST), *18*
  total wake time (TWT), *18*

wake time after sleep-onset (WASO), *18, 23, 52*
sleep spindles, *12*
sleep state mis-perception, *25*
sleepiness, *76, 78*
  see also napping,
  in insomnia, *38*
sleeping pills, *55, 57, 58, 71, 73, 90, 113, 145, 293, 294, 296, 297, 299, 302, 303, 305, 306*
  addiction to, *154*
  and CBT, *297, 299, 303, 305, 306*
  dependence on, *296, 297*
  long-acting and short-acting, *302, 303*
  and persistent insomnia, *294*
  safe withdrawal from, *299, 302, 303, 305, 306*
sleep-onset-latency (SOL), *18, 23, 52*
sleep-related breathing disorder, *151*
snoring, *109, 170, 173, 318, 320*
social and working life, *85, 86*
Spielman, Dr Art, *62, 63, 197*

and model of insomnia development and persistence, *62*
stages of sleep, *9, 12, 13, 15, 18, 19, 20*
  Stage, *3, 9, 12, 19*
  Stage, *3, 9, 12, 19*
  wakefulness (Stage W), *9, 19*
stress, *39, 41, 57, 63, 66, 182, 327, 328*
  and stressors, *49, 148, 150, 155*

T
tables,
  average sleep requirements at different ages, *48*
  bed–sleep connection, strengthening, *204*
  caffeine products that you use, *168*
  CBT program, *96*
  clock-watching, *262*
  diagnosis of insomnia, *52*
  different types of treatment goal, *130*

evaluating thoughts and concerns about insomnia: examples, *161*
evaluating thoughts and concerns about insomnia: worksheet, *161*
giving up trying to sleep, methods for, *255*
other disorders of sleep, *109*
personal sleep history, *103*
putting CBT program into practice, *274*
sleep disorders other than insomnia, *312, 315*
sleep hygiene changes in bedroom environment, *179*
sleeping pills, *302*
temperature (of), *176, 179*
  body, *19, 174*
  room, *172, 174*
thought-evaluation, *163, 247*
  blocking, *248, 250*
  emotions, *227, 228*
  measuring content of, *228, 229, 245*

problem-solving, 223
putting the day to rest, 229, 247, 248
rehearsing and planning, 222, 223
self-awareness, 225
sleeping, 225
thinking, 227
time in bed (TIB), 18, 70, 208, 219, 264
thinking, 222, 253
total sleep time (TST), 18, 46, 48, 208

U

understanding sleep and insomnia, 136, 137, 139, 141, 142, 144, 145, 147, 148, 150, 151, 152, 154, 155, 156, 158, 159, 161, 163
by evaluating your thoughts, 159, 161, 163
sleep quiz for, 139, 141, 142, 144, 145, 147, 148, 150, 151, 152, 154, 155, 156, 158
by using information to change your mind, 158
University of Glasgow Sleep Research Laboratory, 64

V

variations in sleep, 32, 35, 36, 37, 38, 39, 41, 42, 43, 45, 46, 48, 49
see also insomnia, age changes in sleep pattern, 35, 36, 37, 141, 142
good and poor sleepers, 38, 39, 41, 42
individual, 43, 45
and normal range of sleep times, 46, 48
owl and lark tendencies, 45
and sleep deprivation, 42, 43
sleeping across the night, 32, 35
taking naps, 37, 38
see also napping,

W

wake time, 311
after sleep-onset (WASO), 18, 23, 52
total (TWT), 18
waking up briefly, 23, 25
weight changes and effect on sleep, 170